THE ONLINE WORLD OF SURROGACY

Fertility, Reproduction and Sexuality

THE ONLINE WORLD
OF SURROGACY

Zsuzsa Berend

berghahn
NEW YORK · OXFORD
www.berghahnbooks.com

First published in 2016 by

Berghahn Books

www.BerghahnBooks.com

© 2016, 2018 Zsuzsa Berend
First paperback edition published in 2018

Library of Congress Cataloging-in-Publication Data

Names: Berend, Zsuzsa, author.
Title: The online world of surrogacy / Zsuzsa Berend.
Description: New York : Berghahn Books, 2016 | Series: Fertility,
  reproduction and sexuality ; volume 35 | Includes bibliographical
  references and index.
Identifiers: LCCN 2016021756 (print) | ISBN 9781785332746 (hbk:
  alk. paper) | ISBN 9781789200645 (pbk: alk. paper) | ISBN
  9781785332753 (ebook)
Subjects: LCSH: Surrogate mothers—Case studies. | Internet—Social
  aspects. | Human reproductive technology—Social aspects.
Classification: LCC HQ759.5 .B47 2016 | DDC 302.23/1—dc23
LC record available at hbps://lccn.loc.gov/2016021756

British Library Cataloguing in Publication Data

A catalogue record for this book is available from the British Library.

ISBN 978-1-78533-274-6 (hardback)
ISBN 978-1-78920-064-5 (paperback)
ISBN 978-1-78533-275-3 (ebook)

This book is dedicated to the memory of my mother, Rozsa Berger, and to my children, Benjamin and Daniel, without whom this work may have been written more quickly but life would make a lot less sense.

Contents

ACKNOWLEDGMENTS

I wish to thank Rene Almeling, Elijah Anderson, Christopher Colwell, Michael DeLand, Robert Emerson, Alice Goffman, Renee Fox, Jennifer Haylett, Linda Layne, Jody Madeira, Michael Pollak, and Elly Teman for providing very useful comments on some chapters. Rogers Brubaker encouraged this project from the very beginning, and I thank him for believing in it.

Over the years, I often talked to friends about this project. Elijah Anderson, Cesar Ayala, Christopher Colwell, Leslie Dick, Michael DeLand, Michael Pollak, Katya Rice, Christine Schneider, France Winddance Twine, and Joan Waugh heard more about surrogacy than they ever wanted to. I'm grateful to them for listening and also for their assurances that they enjoyed every minute of it. I'm very appreciative of their friendship and the many conversations we had during walks and over wine, and, happily, not only about surrogacy. Very special thanks are due to Elly Teman, whose generous engagement in this project and careful reading and thoughtful comments have been true gifts. I am thankful to Judit Fridli, Eva Havasi, Eva Kerpel, Katalin Koncz, and Andrea Veszits, my friends in Budapest, for their enduring friendship and interest in the project, especially since surrogacy does not translate easily and they have many pressing and dire political issues to worry about in present-day Hungary.

My family deserves special thanks. Ivan Berend and Kati Radics helped me through many bumps during the years this book was in the making, and Dora Gyarmati had faith in my ability to write an even more popular book on surrogacy—maybe next time. Benjamin Brubaker, a budding physicist and brilliant writer, read several chapters and cheerfully corrected punctuation errors and pointed out passages that needed clarification. Daniel Brubaker, more interested in evolutionary biology than third-party reproduction, was convinced that I had already finished this book some years ago, which gave me extra incentive to actually finish it.

Last, but certainly not least, I am appreciative of all the surrogates whose discussions and responses enabled me to think about all these issues.

INTRODUCTION

"Are you still interested in surrogacy?" Lisa asked me in an e-mail in the spring of 2003. "I read your post on SMO, somehow I just came across it now. I also checked the UCLA website just to verify who you say you are, and I'm happy to say that I found you. It makes me feel better giving any information to you." The post Lisa referred to was a short query I had posted earlier on www.surromomsonline.com (SMO), a surrogacy support website, or as it says on its home page, a "virtual meeting ground for the surrogacy community."

I had introduced myself as a sociologist interested in surrogacy and asked women to answer some questions. I was looking to clarify some issues that emerged from reading SMO threads. I wanted to know who these women were, what they thought about being pregnant for someone else, and how they navigated SMO discussions that were both personal and public. I was intrigued by the often intimate tone of SMO communications, especially since women clearly used this public forum to educate people—newbies, intended parents, intended parent hopefuls, and anyone else that happened to be on the site—about surrogacy. I was not the only outsider posting on SMO. Even at the time, but especially over the years, I noticed that a growing number of journalists, documentary film-makers, students, and researchers looked for willing participants for their projects.

Surrogacy has captured the public imagination with its prom-ise—or threat—to transform the most basic of American institu-tions, the family. With the help of a surrogate, infertile heterosexual, older, as well as single people and same-sex couples may realize their dream of parenthood. But surrogacy has also raised questions about relatedness and motherhood, the commodification of life, and the usefulness of surrogacy contracts.[1]

Many of the early critics of surrogacy warned about "reproductive brothels,"[2] the "commodification of motherhood,"[3] and patriarchal control over women.[4] They not only feared but were convinced that financially needy women would be coerced by circumstances and exploited by better educated and more affluent couples. These critics gave fundamentally "normative, indeed political," accounts of social reality.[5] They often referenced patriarchal exploitation and economic pressures but did not take surrogates' experience and perspective into consideration. Yet if we want to understand why this reproductive practice has been growing and evolving, we need to know and appreciate the concerns, experiences, and positions of the surrogates who not only participate in it but actively propagate it. Thus, I am engaging in an "'interpretation,' 'reading,' or 'way of making sense'" of surrogacy.[6]

To be sure, scholars have been making sense of new reproduction and reproductive technologies and practices for decades.[7] Rayna Rapp's questioning of the naturalness of pregnancy, her emphasis on the complexity of women's experience of technology, and her investigation of their narratives of choice informs my work.[8] I share Sarah Franklin and Celia Roberts's approach and goal "to develop a language of social description" that takes into account contested terms, negotiations, and ambivalent and even contradictory responses to reproductive technologies.[9]

I also appreciate their scholarly focus on "a specific technique in a particular country and during a distinct historical period."[10] It is only through careful examination of specific practices and meanings grounded in place and time that we can hope to understand broader issues. Charis Thompson's critique of the argument that medical technology objectifies the patient, depriving her of agency, and her association of agency with "the moral fabric of people's lives" and "locally plausible and enforceable networks of accountability" was also a useful vantage point from which to examine my data.[11]

The past several decades saw an efflorescence of qualitative research on technologies and practices such as in vitro fertilization (IVF), sonogram, amniocentesis, egg and sperm donation, preimplantation genetic testing, and genetic counseling.[12] This scholarship has furthered the understanding not only of the use and meaning of reproductive technologies but also of how new practices "both alter and maintain dominant assumptions and institutions."[13]

My empirical exploration of US surrogacy is thus informed not only by the findings of the large and growing scholarship on reproduction but also by the questions scholars have asked and the perspectives they have taken. My interpretive study follows in the footsteps of the few qualitative explorations of US surrogacy, none of them recent. Helena Ragoné's *Surrogate Motherhood: Conceptions in the Heart,* published in 1994, was the first empirical study of US surrogacy.

Ragoné visited surrogacy programs—at the time eight established programs controlled the surrogacy market—interviewed program directors and staff members, surrogates and intended parents and conducted participant observations over a two-year period. She explored the workings of the programs as well as the feelings, motivations, and expectations of surrogates and couples. She documented how surrogates, with the help of agency personnel and agency-organized support groups, defined surrogacy as a calling rather than a job, as "giving the gift of life" rather than economic exchange. Ragoné analyzed the cultural work the participants engaged in as they reworked kinship concepts, emphasizing intent as the basis of parenthood. However, this cultural work has not revolutionized kinship; rather, it highlighted elements of the practice that are consistent with contemporary middle-class understandings of family relatedness, privileging love, nurture, and commitment.

Elizabeth Roberts's work also explored the empirical reality of surrogacy; she conducted fieldwork and interviews in a California agency. Like Ragoné, Roberts also found that surrogates take pride in their fertility and regard it as an asset and a source of power, and this works to level the socioeconomic difference between them and their couple. Roberts describes surrogates as "strong, independent, self-determined, fertile, and empathic," women who "exert a type of narrative power."[14] Given the nature of my data, "narrative power" is a very fitting concept for surrogates' online stories and communications.

Ragoné's and Roberts's work provide the background for examining continuities and changes in the social and cultural organization of the growing practice of US surrogacy. New technologies and improved success rates of IVF enable new combinations of surrogate and "donated" gametes and even "embryo adoption." The number of agencies has increased exponentially, and lawyers and clinics have entered as reproductive brokers. At the same time, the Internet has become a major forum for both independent matching and information about every aspect of surrogacy, including a growing number of threads (i.e., online discussions on a message board) on the pros and cons of various intermediaries (agencies, lawyers, clinics). As brokers increasingly compete for clients, the Internet has enabled new forms of connections and support for people interested in surrogacy.

Research on surrogacy in other countries provides intriguing empirical comparisons. For example, the inconsistencies of assisted practices in India and the United States give considerable freedom to clinics.[15] In the United States, however, surrogates are generally better educated and have culturally different gender expectations. Thus, they have worked out an informal online repository of knowledge and network of advice that enable them to understand complex and sometimes contradictory information and better navigate the process. Surrogates in both countries make efforts to establish and maintain a relationship with their intended parents, albeit in different, culturally specific ways that also address the different economic options and life situations of surrogates in the two countries.[16]

Elly Teman's ethnography of Israeli surrogacy offers a fascinating comparison.[17] The Israeli and US approaches to surrogacy are in many ways opposites, yet there are some striking similarities between surrogates' conceptualization of the practice. The Israeli state actively supports and tightly controls surrogacy contracts and mandates a rigorous screening process, while US surrogacy is regulated at the state level, if at all, and contracts are often unenforceable.[18]

Teman connects women's narratives to the Israeli sociocultural context and the regulatory practices of the pronatalist state. Israeli medical professionals and the public trivialize gestation in favor of genetics, while in the United States genetics is very often downplayed in comparison to intent, a concept Israelis do not reference. However, both Israeli and American surrogates think of themselves as carriers of the host fetus and often use the same metaphors of "babysitting," "incubating," and "baking." In both countries surrogates embrace the concept of "birthing a mother" and define surrogacy as creating and nurturing not just babies but also parents.

These empirical studies paint a complex picture of the relationships, interests, and emotions of its practitioners. They challenge the binary understanding of surrogacy as either simple commodification, as many feminist critics have framed the issue, or altruism, as journalists increasingly tend to do.[19] In exploring these complexities, I find Viviana Zelizer's "relational work" an illuminating concept to make sense of my data.[20] Zelizer argues that people make considerable efforts to negotiate the meanings of social relations and mark their boundaries, especially when these relations involve both intimacy and economic transactions.[21] We establish meaningful ties to others and carefully distinguish these ties by differentiating the rights, obligations, and transactions that belong to them, marking them with different names and practices of exchange.[22]

I see surrogacy as an instance of an intertwined cultural, emotional, and economic—in other words, *social*—practice whereby people make creative efforts to establish, maintain, negotiate, and transform interpersonal ties of intimacy within a contractual agreement and "engage in the process of differentiating meaningful social relations."[23] This approach shifts the attention from individual actors to interpersonal transactions, the negotiation of relations, and the construction of meaning. The concept of relational work fits well with the interactionist perspective I have adopted for this study. My focus, then, is not on reproductive technologies or the politics of reproduction but on the interactions that create shared understandings, ideas, and desires among the women who assist reproduction.

Building on the above scholarship and, also in each chapter, on a range of sociological, anthropological, and legal scholarship on assisted reproduction, relatedness, contract, money, and gift, I explore the meanings surrogates discursively create on SMO. My research questions address these discursive interactions or interactive discourses that shape the social and emotional organization of assisted reproduction.[24] Women have been jointly working out what it means to be a surrogate and what kinds of behaviors are consistent with their dream of "giving the gift of life."

Marcia Inhorn and Daphna Birenbaum-Carmeli argued, "It is always important to keep the problem of infertility in clear view when discussing ARTs."[25] US surrogates do not let the researcher forget this, and their frequent and elaborate discussions of infertility and its pain also remind us that the definition of infertility is very much local. The operative definition of infertility on SMO is inability to have children even past childbearing age or to have as many children as one would like. This definition shapes surrogates' empathy and informs their determination to "help couples," whether childless, or gay, or past childbearing age, or "not done with their family."

I situate my investigation in the context of larger sociocultural ideas and practices concerning family, parenthood, money, gift, and technology in the United States. My data point to a collective, Internet-based effort to create surrogates as well as surrogacy, an endeavor that has its rules, rituals, and rewards that are independent of individual biographies. Surrogates' accounts are compelling and fascinating cases of individual agency, situated in and invigorated as well as tempered by what Goffman called "interaction ritual."[26]

I began this project in a somewhat unusual way. My earlier research was on nineteenth-century unmarried women and their notions of love, duty, work, money, and family. Then I moved to Los Angeles, woefully far from my beloved archives in Massachusetts, and with two young children I knew I would not be able to bridge the distance. A few years later I started teaching a lecture course, the Sociology of the Family, and assigned parts of Helena Ragoné's book on surrogacy. One of the students in that class chose to do a paper on surrogacy, using SMO as her source of data. In order to be able to give her advice, I logged on. I became intrigued with online discussions; I saw this as a brave new frontier. The online discussions intrigued me no less than the letters and diaries I had researched in the past; deciphering both required close attention to detail and meaning. SMO threads invoked the importance of family, referenced self-sacrifice and vocation; these were priorities and concepts that were familiar from my previous research.

My reading of SMO threads resonated with many of Ragoné's arguments about the conceptualization of surrogacy. Nevertheless, there were major differences. In Ragoné's study, surrogacy agencies played a central role in framing the meaning of surrogacy and mediating interactions, while on SMO women communicated with one another and offered advice without institutional mediation. This was a self-regulating group; surrogates were taking charge of the process in many ways, advocating surrogacy and policing the website.[27]

This new type of social control was intriguing, and I became interested in the collective emotional and relational work, the joint negotiations, and the meaning making surrogates engaged in on SMO. Reading surrogates' discussions convinced me that these women were creative players in a new social situation; online interactions shape and coordinate their thinking about the problems and questions that arise. Discussions reveal joint efforts to negotiate and define the balance between selflessness and self-protection, between giving and receiving. Communications revolve around taking charge of the process and serve as both learning tools and vehicles of support and appreciation. Women collectively strive to affirm the value of helping behavior and normalize surrogacy and the emotions it gives rise to. They learn to deal with disappointments and to be "the better person" and define what it means to be a good surrogate.

By focusing on the dynamic and formative nature of SMO communications I am by no means trying to take away from the uniqueness of women's stories. Rather, my argument emphasizes the creative process whereby shared understandings and definitions emerge from their discussions.

The relatively new practice of surrogacy has been evolving in front of our eyes and offers us insights into how people make sense of what they do as they chart new territories. Attention to discussions and negotiated meanings among surrogates and participating intended parents reveal the moral project they are engaged in; good and bad, appropriate and inappropriate, are defined by the group. Empirical exploration of these negotiations enables us to ask better questions about the intersection of market and nonmarket activities, of monetary and intimate relationships in surrogacy and beyond. Thus, rather than rehearsing the old and not particularly fruitful questions about the moral perils or possible economic benefits of commodification or debating whether certain things should be kept out of the reach of the market, we may turn our attention to what Fourcade and Healy call "moralized markets."[28] "How gift and market exchange relate to moral worth is, ultimately, an empirical question," and this is the question that I take up in my research.[29]

Lisa, the surrogate who contacted me to ask if I was still interested in surrogacy, soon became my key informant. She told me her unfolding story and answered the many questions that SMO threads raised for me. She was a working divorced mother of two teenagers; she had given birth to twins in January 2003 as a traditional surrogate (TS). Traditional surrogates are artificially inseminated, either at the doctor's office or at home, and are genetically related to the baby. By the time she began writing to me Lisa was actively looking for new intended parents, commonly known as IPs, that is, a couple to carry a baby for.[30] Even though Lisa, like most surrogates, was asking for compensation, she was also hoping to find her "perfect match." This did not surprise me because I had already noticed the prevalence of the language of love ("I fell in love with this couple" and "we clicked right away") in surrogates' writings.

What did surprise me, however, was Lisa's determination to find a new couple so soon after the birth of twins; the second twin's birth was by C-section and Lisa was unhappy about that. Initially, she wanted to do another traditional surrogacy, but by September she was open to a gestational "journey." Gestational surrogates are not genetically related to the fetus they carry.[31] They go through an "embryo transfer" procedure in which the fertilized eggs are put in a plastic catheter, which is placed near the top of the uterus. The placement is guided by ultrasound imaging and once the catheter is in place, the embryos are expelled into the uterus.

Gestational surrogates all take Lupron, a hormone to regulate their menstrual cycle, four to five weeks before the transfer. Just before and after the transfer gestational surrogates are also on estrogen and progesterone, hormone pills and injections, to thicken the uterine lining. Some take aspirin and antibiotics, and even steroids, for a while. They are on medication for twelve to sixteen weeks if the transfer is successful but for a minimum of two weeks until the blood test result (and continue if it is positive). Since transfers are often unsuccessful, gestational surrogates frequently undergo several cycles with the same or very similar medical protocol each time.

"I'm excited to get started on a new journey as this is important for me to do and I don't want to 'run out of time' to be able to do it. My body is only good for so long and I sure wish I'd known about it much earlier . . . so I could do this many times," Lisa wrote in the fall of 2003. This desire was not uncommon among surrogates on SMO, who joke that surrogacy contracts should include the following: "WARNING: Helping others create families via surrogacy may be addictive. Please plan on having 10+ years available for future journeys." In October Lisa seemed to have found her dream couple. The first phone call went well. "We talked about 1.5 hours . . . about EVERYTHING and we actually get along better than me and my previous IM [intended mother]! It was like it was meant to be." When surrogates "click" or "hit it off" with a couple, their online posts often sound like Lisa's account. When this is not the case, the advice on SMO is likely to be "don't settle for something like this if you don't want to. . . . there's always something perfect out there waiting."

Finding IPs can be a drawn-out and complex procedure. Women research agencies and wait to be matched. With the Internet playing an increasingly important role in the matching process, independent arrangements ("going indy," i.e., without an agency) are on the rise. The parties advertise on sites like SMO, respond to advertisements, and negotiate personal compatibility as well as financial and contractual issues. Lisa described the process in a long e-mail to me. "When my agency was having difficulty matching me, I took it upon myself to place an ad on SMO. After placing my ad, I responded to multiple ads in order to get my name out there and to see if I connected with anyone, etc. Corresponding between multiple PIPs [potential intended parents] is normal." When I noted that the selection process seemed more intricate than online dating, she agreed, "haha, well, I've tried that and it is similar in most ways, but you talk about babies, not dating!!" My idea for this comparison came from the numerous posts I had read in which surrogates liken surrogacy to romantic relationships.

The match about which Lisa was so enthusiastic fell through for financial reasons. "They determined that 'in case I was put on bedrest' they could not afford to pay my net wages. . . . They did not have the 'extras' for maternity clothes, expenses, multiple fee, c-section fee, etc. That all could potentially increase the fee over $10K," Lisa wrote. By December 2003, she had talked to a number of agencies, couples, and single men. The e-mails that followed betrayed Lisa's frustration. Then she wrote me about a failed home insemination. I asked who the couple was. "The couple is the same couple who didn't have money. I dropped a lot of fees/extras and have extended the time to pay out for 6 months after delivery! The IM and I have such a connection, I just couldn't walk away."

Lisa decided to forgo her lost wages and life insurance requests. "I have such a connection with my IM that I couldn't see doing this for anyone else." But after the failed attempt, there were no more tries. The intended father had reservations and did not want to continue. Lisa explained that she had tried to change their minds because she was "concerned for the out-of-pocket $$ they have already spent and wanted them to at least try. I don't think they will. For whatever reasons, IF [intended father] thinks he's "cheating" on IM," Lisa told me. Surrogates are not the only ones who borrow from the language of love.

Lisa, who was in her midthirties and impatient to find new IPs, continued to look for a match both with and without agency help. She lives in a "surrogacy-unfriendly" state and that was a hindrance.[32] Finally, in the fall of 2004, Lisa was matched through an agency as a gestational surrogate. The IPs were an older couple in a second marriage; the IM had a grown son from her first marriage, but her husband had no children. They were using an egg donor and the husband's sperm. Lisa had two fertilized eggs transferred at the beginning of October. At the end of October the ultrasound showed one sack with a yoke and fetal pole (i.e., one of the fertilized eggs implanted), but it was too early for the heartbeat.

In November Lisa miscarried. However, it was not until January 2006 that, in an answer to my question about pregnancy loss, she told me more about that miscarriage: "as far as any support from my IPs prior, during or after the miscarriage, there was NONE.

Not a call to see how I was doing, how am I feeling, am I in pain (? what? Pain during a miscarriage? How about working an 8 hour day in a law firm DURING a miscarriage?? I did it.) They grieved, yet showed me no comfort during that time and then they pulled away completely and I had no idea as to what they were thinking or anything. They even talked to the RE [reproductive endocrinologist] and were told that I had nothing to do with it, it wasn't my fault, it just quit growing for some reason. I did everything I was supposed to do. . . . They still didn't talk to me for a while."

Lisa's experience is similar to that of many surrogates whose stories I read on SMO. Women express anxiety and often confess to feeling responsible for crashing the couple's hopes, although not for the miscarriage itself. And, most often, they are alone with their pain and anxiety. "I felt the same way as you," one surrogate on SMO comforted another who felt lonely after her miscarriage, "that there wasn't really anyone around, or any of my family or friends who really understood how I was feeling. Even my IM; because she was feeling her own feelings and although we are in this together, we have different emotions and are coming from different angles. It is our bodies who had to go through all of this."

But like this surrogate, Lisa was eager to try again for the same couple. By the spring of 2005 Lisa was pregnant with twins but soon "lost one of the twins." She was realistic about the benefits of being pregnant with a singleton but felt bad for her couple. Her IM was "very upset." As the pregnancy progressed, Lisa experienced serious swelling in her feet and often had to call in sick. In October, she delivered by C-section, something she was hoping to avoid. A bad infection set in soon after she was released from the hospital. She had a very high fever and had to go to the emergency room. She also developed high blood pressure.

This was not the only hardship Lisa had to endure. Her surrogacy contract did not cover all her lost wages. "I've lost so much money with this surrogacy and having my lost wages capped because no one told me disability only paid $1700 per month, only half of what I was normally making!" She confessed that she lost more money on this surrogacy than on her first one. And because she was on sick leave more than her boss tolerated, she lost her job.

When I pressed Lisa, she admitted that she had told her IM about her predicament. "I emailed my IM and told her I'd lost my job and I've yet to hear back from her about it. I've been emailing about 'other' things with her but no comment on this. I guess it's my responsibility to find a job (of course it is) and it must be my fault too? *sigh* Of course, I wouldn't have lost it had I NOT been prego so that's the part that kills me."

She regularly received pictures of her "surrobaby," which she promptly forwarded to her surrogate friends, and to me. After I sent her a link about a surrogate who was not paid after a miscarriage because of the way the contract was phrased, Lisa agreed that "it's really upsetting to read threads like that but the responsibility falls on the surrogate to cover her own ass . . . this one failed, as I did. Next time, she'll be a bit smarter. Like I will be." Lisa was a realist, most of the time. However, things did not work out well for her. She had found several temporary and part-time jobs and was still looking for a permanent one when I e-mailed with her last. Lisa's son, then nineteen years old, was killed in a hit-and-run accident in the fall of 2007. I received Lisa's group e-mails about this and about the funeral, but she never again corresponded with me after this tragedy. I continued to see her occasional posts on SMO for a while, but then she disappeared from there, too.

My initial curiosity coupled with Lisa's frequent e-mails drew me deep into this project, and I found myself logging on to SMO to see "what my surrros were doing." There were many stories similar to Lisa's. Women were eager to embark on a surrogate "journey," often exploring both agency and independent matching options. They enthusiastically posted about the intended parents they "clicked with," the vicissitudes of the contract negotiations, and their pregnancies and birth stories; they made financial and other compromises and adjustments to carry a baby for someone else. They happily shared stories of updates from former IPs and posted photos of flowers and other gifts they received from their couple. There were also many anguished accounts of miscarriages, feelings of guilt for letting their couple down, and complaints about the lack of support and empathy from intended parents. Some women, like Lisa, have lost money or their job. And whether the journey went well or not, many surrogates wrote of their resolve to do it again.

As I immersed myself in SMO discussions I realized that this forum was by no means simply a meeting place for women who shared the same "dream to help infertile couples." SMO threads teach women what to expect, want, and dream of. Surrogates often reference the same dream: seeing the IPs' faces and the tears in their eyes as they hold their baby after birth. This may be the single most powerful image of surrogacy, and one that continues to exercise enormous power over newcomers and old-timers alike. The online medium enables the image to be clearly formulated through countless posts describing the expectation of tears and smiles at the moment of the ultimate giving.

Lisa and most of the women who have posted on SMO over the years actively pursue surrogacy, collect information, go through hardships, and increasingly applaud stories that project independence and self-sufficiency. They increasingly think of surrogacy as a purposeful, goal-oriented series of actions that is in many ways its own reward. One of the moderators on SMO wrote with the authority of seniority, "You can do anything that you really want to do, there are no limits with smart and educated women."

This sounds very much like the "myriad of micropractices" that Sawicki suggested we should describe and analyze in order to understand reproductive technology as "neither inherently liberating nor repressive," and whose "meaning derives from the social and political context in which it is embedded."[33] The ways in which participants make sense of assisted reproduction within specific sociocultural contexts is not a simple matter; social actors "can understand an interaction in different, and conflicting, ways."[34] This book is an exploration of such meaning-creating practices.

Overview of the book

In Chapter 1, "The Virtual Meeting Ground for Real People," I introduce SMO, discuss its organization and membership, and describe my methods.

Chapter 2, "Journey," describes the "journey of shared love" that ideally starts with a feeling of chemistry between the surrogate and the intended parents. Surrogates do not embark on this journey alone and husbands' support is essential. Women also work out the relationship to the fetus they carry and redefine relatedness in creative ways. The love rhetoric reframes commercial surrogacy as an intimate relationship with the intended parents. Thus, surrogates mourn reproductive losses, whether they are failed conceptions or miscarriages, which represent the loss of their own surrogacy dreams and also mobilize women to show their empathy for their couples. Love is the logical antithesis of commodification; women insist that there is no full compensation for this kind of giving. This rendering of surrogacy counters the stigma of "baby production"; paradoxically, though, framing surrogacy as a selfless "labor of love" not only enables but also encourages women to repeatedly carry babies for others.

Chapter 3, "Contract," gives a detailed description and analysis of contract negotiations as revealed by SMO posts. The currency evoked in these discussions is both monetary fees and moral worth. Contrary to most legal theories, surrogates and intended parents often do not see the contract the same way and are not always trying to achieve the same goals. Surrogates' view, not explored by legal scholars, that the contract is the basis of the social relationship with IPs is consequential for surrogacy outcomes. Surrogates are also keenly aware of the limitations of the contract in regulating meaningful relationships; friendship is real if it is freely given.

Chapter 4, "Money," takes up the financial side of surrogacy, which has important both practical and symbolic significance. Surrogates generally want to save money for their intended parents and often compromise on fees for the "right couple." The numerous discussions and stories reveal rich layers of symbolic meanings. Monetary dealings are always understood in the context of the relationship with IPs. Discussions also show that women carefully match the various monetary transactions with their interpretation of the relationship.

Chapter 5, "Gift," investigates the actual and symbolic gifting practices between surrogates and their couple and the centrality of gift giving in surrogates' definition of surrogacy. Surrogates often receive tangible gifts at various times during the journey and also intangible gifts like time, attention, and trust. Their countergifts include efforts to allow couples to experience "their pregnancy" as well as presents that mark memorable occasions. SMO discussions reveal a deep desire to transform the surrogate journey into a mutual gift-giving relationship in which tangible and intangible gifts flow back and forth.

Finally, "Conclusion" sums up the major findings and highlights the discursive creation of the online world of surrogacy and the ways in which surrogates turn jointly negotiated understandings into platforms for actions. It offers some thoughts about the ways in which surrogates' self-organizational, emotional, and cultural work shape both the market in third-party reproduction and its moral meaning. It also offers some thoughts on the generalizability of these findings for the interrelated nature of gift and market in postindustrial societies.

Notes

1. Most recently, France Winddance Twine asked some of these questions in a comparative context. FW Twine, *Outsourcing the Womb: Race, Class and Gestational Surrogacy in a Global Market* (New York: Routledge, 2015).
2. Gena Corea, *The Mother Machine: Reproductive Technologies from Artificial Insemination to Artificial Wombs* (New York: Harper & Row, 1985); Andrea Dworkin, *Right-Wing Women* (London: Women's Press, 1987).
3. Elizabeth S. Anderson, "Is Women's Labor a Commodity?" *Philosophy and Public Affairs* 19, no. 1 (1990): 71–92; Barbara Katz Rothman, "Comment on Harrison: The Commodification of Motherhood," *Gender and Society* 1, no. 3 (1987): 312–16; Martha A. Field, *Surrogate Motherhood* (Cambridge, MA: Harvard University Press, 1988), 25–32.
4. Dworkin, *Right-Wing Women*; Christine Overall, *Ethics and Human Reproduction: A Feminist Analysis* (Boston: Allen and Unwin, 1987).
5. Gabriel Abend, "The Meaning of 'Theory,'" *Sociological Theory* 26, no. 2 (2008): 180.
6. Ibid.,178.
7. E.g., Gay Becker, *The Elusive Embryo: How Women and Men Approach New Reproductive Technologies* (Berkeley: University of California Press, 2000); Faye D. Ginsburg and Rayna Rapp, *Conceiving the New World Order: The Global Politics of Reproduction* (Berkeley: University of California Press, 1995); Susan Markens, *Surrogate Motherhood and the Politics of Reproduction* (Berkeley: University of California Press, 2007).
8. Rayna Rapp, *Testing Women, Testing the Fetus. The Social Impact of Amniocentesis in America* (New York: Routledge, 1999).
9. Sarah Franklin and Cecil Roberts, *Born and Made: An Ethnography of Preimplantation Genetic Diagnosis* (Princeton: Princeton University Press, 2006), 11.
10. Ibid., xv.
11. Charis Thompson, *Making Parents. The Ontological Choreography of Reproductive Technologies* (Cambridge, MA: MIT Press, 2005), 181.
12. E.g., Rene Almeling, *Sex Cells: The Medical Market for Eggs and Sperm* (Berkeley: University of California Press, 2011); Marcia C. Inhorn, *Local Babies, Global Science: Gender, Religion, and in Vitro Fertilization in Egypt* (New York: Routledge, 2003); Susan Markens, Carole H. Browner, and H. Mabel Preloran, "Interrogating the Dynamics between Power, Knowledge and Pregnant Bodies in Amniocentesis Decision Making," *Sociology of Health & Illness* 32, no. 1 (2010): 37–56; Lisa Meryn Mitchell, *Baby's First Picture: Ultrasound and the Politics of Fetal Subjects* (Toronto: University of Toronto Press, 2001); Margarete Sandelowski, *With Child in Mind: Studies of the Personal Encounter with Infertility* (Philadelphia: University of Pennsylvania Press, 1993); Janelle S. Taylor, *The Public Life of the Fetal Sonogram: Technology, Consumption, and the Politics of Reproduction* (New Brunswick, NJ: Rutgers University Press, 2008).

13. Laura Mamo, *Queering Reproduction. Achieving Pregnancy in the Age of Technoscience* (Durham: Duke University Press, 2007), 5.
14. Elizabeth F.S. Roberts, "Examining Surrogacy Discourses between Feminine Power and Exploitation," in *Small Wars: The Cultural Politics of Childhood,* ed. N. Scheper-Hughes and C. Sargent (Berkeley: University of California Press, 1998), 108.
15. Kalindi Vora, "Potential, Risk, and Return in Transnational Indian Gestational Surrogacy," *Current Anthropology* 54, no. S7 (2013): S97–S106.
16. Ibid.; also Amrita Pande, *Wombs in Labor: Transnational Commercial Surrogacy in India* (New York: Columbia University Press, 2014); Sharmila Rudrappa, "India's Reproductive Assembly Line," *Contexts* 11, no. 2 (2012): 22–27.
17. Elly Teman, *Birthing a Mother: The Surrogate Body and the Pregnant Self* (Berkeley: University of California Press, 2010).
18. Diane Hinson and Maureen McBrian, "Surrogacy across America," accessed 15 September 2013, http://claradoc.gpa.free.fr/doc/431.pdf.
19. Susan Markens, "The Global Reproductive Health Market: U.S. Media Framings and Public Discourses about Transnational Surrogacy," *Social Science & Medicine* 74, no. 11 (2012): 1745–53.
20. Viviana A. Zelizer, *The Purchase of Intimacy* (Princeton, NJ: Princeton University Press, 2005), 35.
21. Ibid., 34–35.
22. Ibid., 32–33.
23. Viviana A. Zelizer, "How I Became a Relational Economic Sociologists and What Does That Mean?" *Politics & Society* 40, no. 2 (2012): 146.
24. Zelizer's point that "interaction . . . produces structure" is relevant here. Zelizer, "Relational Economic Sociologist,"150.
25. Marcia C. Inhorn and Daphna Birenbaum-Carmeli, "Assisted Reproductive Technologies and Cultural Change," *Annual Review of Anthropology* 37 (2008): 179. Also see Marcia Inhorn and Frank van Balen, eds., *Infertility around the Globe. New Thinking on Childlessness, Gender, and Reproductive Technologies* (Berkeley: University of California Press, 2002).
26. Erving Goffman, *Interaction Ritual: Essays on Face-to-Face Behavior* (New York: Pantheon Books, 1967). While Goffman's subtitle is "Face-to-Face Behavior," he argues that everyone "lives in a world of social encounters" involving the person "in face-to-face or mediated contact with other participants" (ibid., 5). Mediated interactions involve fewer senses, thus fewer cues, but my findings show that women on SMO utilize symbolic signals like emoticons, abbreviations, and internal references, adding nuance to the verbal repertoire.
27. Policing practices by members includes identifying inconsistencies in posts, probing into suspicious-sounding stories, and confronting members who breach stated or tacit rules of engagement.
28. Marion Fourcade and Kieran Healy, "Moral Views of Market Society," *Annual Review of Sociology* 33 (2007): 299.

29. Ibid., 301.

30. "Commissioning couple" is a term often used by legal and feminist scholars but never by surrogates or intended parents on SMO. My findings show that SMO-ers do not think about surrogacy as commission or IPs as commissioning.

31. Gestational surrogacy, often using "donor" gametes, has become vastly more common; according to some questionable estimates, it accounts for 95 percent of commercial surrogacy arrangements. This statistic has been cited by several legal scholars who reference one other. Mark Strasser's recent piece cites a 2011 paper that in turn cites a 2007 article (Strasser, Mark. "Tradition Surrogacy Contracts, Partial Enforcement, and the Challenge for Family Law." *Journal of Health Care Law & Policy*, 18 (2015): 85-113). At the end of the reference chain, I found the original source, RESOLVE fact sheet #56. This fact sheet, "could not be found" on RESOLVE's website although a RESOLVE web page on surrogacy contains a link to it: http://familybuilding.resolve.org/site/PageServer?pagename=cop_eaotpo_srgcy&printer_friendly=1. A 2003 estimate claimed that more than 50 percent of surrogates have been gestational since 1994 (http://www.encyclopedia.com/topic/surrogate_mother.aspx). The basis of these estimates is the number of clinics that work with traditional surrogates. The picture is further complicated by the inconsistent, state-by-state regulation; some states ban traditional surrogacy, some others ban all compensated surrogacy, and some do not regulate it. See http://creativefamilyconnections.com/wp-content/uploads/2013/12/FamilyAdvocateSurrogacyAcrossAmerica.pdf. But we cannot really know; assisted practices are not recorded on birth certificates. Agencies have no reporting obligation but would be unable to accurately report in any event because surrogates and intended parents (IPs) frequently match independently online or through lawyers, as SMO evidence indicates. Also, many traditional surrogates do home inseminations to save money for their couple and thus leave no official trail. The Council for Responsible Genetics estimated that gestational surrogacy grew by 89 percent between 2004 and 2008, resulting in 5,238 babies. However, the Centers for Disease Control and Prevention (CDC) collects statistics on IVF cycles rather than individual cases. The CDC's data collection of assisted reproductive technologies (ART) has been evolving since 1996, and the National ART Surveillance System was launched in 2006. The 2012 ART National Summary Report states, "Gestational carriers were used in about 1% of ART cycles using fresh nondonor" eggs and embryos (see http://www.cdc.gov/art/pdf/2012-report/national-summary/art_2012_national_summary_report.pdf). Donor eggs and frozen embryo transfer cycles are not included in any statistics even though these are empirically well documented, common practices.

32. Eleven states—the surrogacy-unfriendly ones—prohibit all or most surrogate agreements. There are many regulatory loopholes and gray areas, but living in a surrogate-unfriendly state makes the arrangement more complicated. See Hinson and McBrian, "Surrogacy across America."
33. Jana Sawicki, *Disciplining Foucault: Feminism, Power, and the Body* (New York: Routledge, 1991), 81.
34. Margaret Jane Radin, *Contested Commodities: The Trouble with Trade in Sex, Children, Body Parts, and Other Things* (Cambridge, MA: Harvard University Press, 1996), 103.

Chapter 1

THE VIRTUAL MEETING GROUND
FOR REAL PEOPLE

The site: "our 'world'"

SMO

S MO is the largest moderated[1] public surrogacy website in the
United States. It calls itself "the virtual meeting ground" for
people interested in surrogacy-related issues; it had around thirty
thousand members (surrogates and intended parents) when I finished data collection,[2] up from around eight hundred in 2002, and
it contained more than 100,000 threads and more than one million
posts. Founded in 1997 and operated by surrogates, this website
is a major source of information and support that guides women's
choices and decisions. SMO is also an exceptionally rich source of
data for research purposes. Women discuss both surrogacy- and
non–surrogacy-related events and problems. The message boards
are divided into seven forums: announcements, general, our journeys, international, miscellaneous, technical issues, and archives.[3]
Overall, there are close to thirty strictly surrogacy-related subforums where women post stories, questions, information, and advice
and where they support and criticize one another.

Members have usernames, and once registered, they are not
allowed to change it or register under a different name. Newcomers ("newbies")[4] have to go through a moderation period, which
is designed to screen out spam, troublemakers, and banned former
members. During this time their posts appear with some delay
because they have to be approved by moderators or the owner of

the site. After they have posted twenty to thirty times and spent a month or two on SMO, the moderation is lifted, although they are still "new users" until one hundred posts or six months after joining.

Once off moderation, women are able to post without delay, e-mail directly, and make a "siggy" or ask someone to make one for them. Siggys are little signature boxes with various, often seasonal, designs, for example cobwebs or witches around Halloween, snowy landscape or Santa Claus around Christmas, and a variety of other designs (flowers, photographs of surrogate and her family, etc.). Siggys often contain the member's first name and marital, mother-hood, and surrogate status and sometimes include the husband's, children's and "surrobabies'" names or initials as well as intended parents' (IPs) initials.

Occasionally, surrogates include a short description to signal emotional connection to some of these people, for example, "wife to the love of my life," "mommy to 3 rugrats," or "GS [gestational surrogate] to amazing IPs." A siggy may be simple: "Wife, mother, optimistic GS" or contain more information: "Kathy, DW [darling wife] to John, mother to 4, GSx3" or "Betty, wife to my soulmate, mother to Ashley, Brittany, and Matt, GSx1for M&T, GSx2 twins for super IFs [intended fathers]." Because women periodically change their siggy design, and because some designs, especially the seasonal ones, are very popular, it is hard to tell who is who at a glance. User-names are unique, although for an outsider "mommyfortwo" may look confusingly similar to 'mommytofour." Members completely immersed in the life of SMO address one another by first name in their replies, even when neither the siggy nor the username reveals it, testifying to their familiarity with one another.[5]

Posts contain information about the date of joining SMO, loca-tion, and number of posts. Some members indicate the city they live in, others only the state, and some playfully list "lalaland," "mommyland," "in the face!" or "wouldn't you want to know?"[6] It is impossible to have meaningful statistics about membership or number of surrogacies, but date of membership and information contained in siggys indicate that many women stay on the boards for years, often doing several surrogacies. To be sure, we cannot know how many women are on the boards for only a short time; what we see is the interactions among those who participate in the discussions. There is no way to estimate what proportion of SMO members regularly engages in discussions, although one can tell how active individual users are from the number of their posts. The more vocal women reach a thousand posts or more a year, although there is great variation.

During my decade of reading on SMO, a few hundred views and five to fifteen replies to a post was typical, although contentious or highly relevant threads got a lot more. Replies were usually between four and ten percent of all views. Once in a while women started a thread about their "SMO addiction," in which many "confess" to not posting much but "checking SMO every five minutes," although Facebook groups were becoming more prominent the last few years.[7]

The interacting group

The interacting SMO group consisted of mostly surrogates, some new and former intended mothers (IMs), and a very few gay intended fathers. Gay IFs received a warm welcome on SMO, but only a couple of them entered into discussions with any regularity. Former IMs, some of whom posted regularly, enjoyed a privileged position. These IMs no longer needed advice and stayed on SMO because they wanted to contribute.[8] Surrogates almost never took issue with these IMs' posts; their opinions and views were highly valued and respected. Other IMs were treated with respect and given the benefit of the doubt but were not immune to criticism, especially when they sounded bitter or demanding.

On the whole, surrogates criticized one another much more than they criticized IMs. Anyone who was not informed or resilient enough or was too "whiney" could face sharp comments, but much depended on context. Women responded critically or even flippantly to ill-informed newbies but also often gave advice and encouraged them to do more research. In general, responses to any question or story very much depended on how the self and the problems were presented: clueless, demanding, self-righteous, self-pitying, and accusatory posts tended to get more and sharper criticism and less sympathy.

After reading discussions on SMO for a while I thought of Howard Becker's simple but brilliant assertion: "Seeing things as the product of people doing things together makes a lot of other views less plausible and less interesting."[9] Surrogates often say that they "could not have done it" without SMO or that they would not have done more than one "journey."[10] These statements may, of course, be interpreted as fairly standard expressions of appreciation for support and advice. But they also illuminate the simple fact that women's conversations and debates on SMO constitute joint activity. Outcomes—shared assumptions and understandings, agreed-upon or contested definitions, learning curves—are the product of women doing things together on SMO.

SMO membership consists of "newbies," "experienced," and "retired" surrogates. These are SMO-ers' own terms, as is "SMO-er." Newbies who introduced themselves on the boards were most often new to surrogacy, although some were new to SMO but not to surrogacy. They were generally warmly greeted and encouraged to ask questions. Ginny, a two-time surrogate, posted several welcoming messages to newbies as well as the following advice:

> If you have questions and are afraid of backlash, find someone to answer off the boards. I will offer my e-mail addy to you. I know sometimes you can't e-mail through the boards until you've been here a while. If you don't think I'm the one you want to talk to I would still be willing to help you reach out to the one you think you might connect with. I might even be able to figure out for you who might be your "ideal" buddy. There is nothing wrong with asking questions on the board since that's what it's here for. However sometimes that doesn't go well for various reasons. If you are just kind of shy maybe you're just afraid to put yourself out there. Anyway, most of us really do want to help. Please keep in mind that if you truly want help, it might not come in the form of what you want to hear. If you only want to hear whatever you want, then please re-evaluate your "calling" to be a surro. If you can take the bad with the good then please jump at the chance. I know there have been attempts at mentoring on here before but I thought it would be a good idea to bring it up again.[11]

This post captures the spirit of SMO by spelling out the rules of engagement—newbies are welcome and gladly mentored if they are willing to listen and learn—yet acknowledges that mentoring is not always gentle. Newbies who do their research were more favorably received than ones who "could have found the answers through searching the site." But displaying too much knowledge is not always good, and newbies who post too frequently tended to be criticized:

> As far as being a "newbie" goes: I don't think most people here care how long you have been a member or how many posts you have (very generally speaking.) The problem arises when you have a member here for two months with a thousand posts to their name, and they act like they know it all. Just because you post on every thread out there to up your count doesn't make you a veteran member.

Veteran status had to be earned; there are no shortcuts to experience or to respect.

Newbies were sometimes made fun of when their questions or stories were not all that clearly articulated. "I'm always confused when newbies come on and post random things," complained one of the experienced surrogates. Veterans of the boards agreed on a newbie code of conduct: "newbies need to just go ahead and ask the ? that they want and need answers to and participate in threads if they see fit. Just be ready to take others' 'opinions.'" Experienced surrogates often cautioned newbies, reminding them how much they still need to learn about being an SMO-er: "Oh, this is a really controversial topic and I don't think you just want to jump in like this!" New members were sometimes chastised, as the following newbie who got into a heated argument with an "experienced" member was: "Ok, do you really want to get in a pissing match with Vic? That's not a good idea. Seriously if I were you, I'd call it a day and just knock it off. Acting like an *** here is never a good idea for a newbie. Not trying to be a rude b**ch or anything, I'm just letting you know up front."

Newcomers were expected to not complain about the responses they received; they were expected to "take it" and learn to conform to group norms. My findings are similar to Kendall's, who, in her work on a multiuser dungeon game that was mainly a "social meeting place," demonstrated that participants consider continuity of group norms important.[12] However, norms are revealed through violations, as we saw in the above passage when a newbie was chastised for taking issue with Vic.

Newbies earned respect by "doing their homework," asking informed questions, taking advice and "opinion" without "an attitude," showing restraint in their communications, and acknowledging their limited experience. When a newbie reported that she had made some mistakes and suffered the consequences, she got the following reply: "I am so sorry to hear you are hurt. . . . But unfortunately these are things that some of the members here have tried to tell ALL new surrogates. I am not saying I told you so by any means but at the same time I just wish newbies would take a step back and really take some of the advice that is given."

The next response was similar: "It's hard for us experienced surrogates to see situations like yours where we KNOW how it will end but people are in too much of a rush to get pregnant that they pay no heed to those trying to help them and advising them to slow down." The newbie was appropriately humbled and also gracious:

"Thanks [ladies] for not saying I told you so but many people here were right that we needed to slow the process way down. I willingly admit that and wish that I had listened to the advice that I was given. I take full responsibility for that. :(" The posts that followed were all sympathetic and wished her all the best. This is the newbie attitude experienced members appreciate, and Ella, the voice of reason, summed it up: "You have learned, and are sharing your knowledge."

Those who left SMO after one surrogacy usually did so quietly, although women who had a very bad surrogacy experience sometimes explained their departure. More outspoken were those who were forced to "retire," usually for medical reasons. These women usually had a hard time becoming reconciled to the end of their surrogacy years and looked for support on the boards. The most frequently offered consolation resonated the most with women: "Realize that you will always be a surrogate even if you are done carrying. Those children that you carried are on this earth with your help, and nothing can take that from you." Retired surrogates usually left the boards once they no longer generated new stories, although many stayed on for a while to advise others, voice opinions, and level criticism or offer support.

One such woman, Ella, managed to not only stay on the boards but also participate in most discussions for more than six years; she carved out a space for herself as the voice of reason and wisdom. She offered short but to-the-point opinions and advice in a range of threads. She was not overly committed to any ideology and was evenhanded in her responses. She "called it as she saw it" and was a little vulgar at times, and although she often referenced her disappointing journey she was not too bitter. She embodied the SMO contention—which she helped to solidify—that in the end a surrogate who was let down or betrayed by her IPs can be "the better person."[13] She often had the last word in discussions; no one openly challenged her views and many enthusiastically seconded her opinion and advice, and even quoted her in their posts. No one else managed to establish this kind of a position, but many wondered about their role on the boards once they retired:

> Do you ever question what your role on SMO is? . . . I have been on SMO for a little over 3 years now. I have given birth to 2 beautiful children, and have helped make 2 sets of IPs parents (which I am very proud of). But as I sit here 4 months PP [postpartum] from delivering my last surrobabe, I wonder what keeps me coming back

to SMO. Is it that surrogacy has been such a major part of my life for 3 years? It seems lately all I do on SMO is make siggys, post some good deals I come across, and occasional comment on a belly pic. Do I still have a place here. . . . I don't know what the future holds for me in terms of another journey. Does anyone else have these feelings?

Ella was quick to join this discussion: "I'll stay until I feel I can no longer offer anything of value. I wish there was someone to yell at ME when I was new and I pointed out things which were red flags. I hope to be that person and prevent someone from making mistakes I made." Lisa told me about this kind of participation by retired or semiretired surrogates: "One of the moderators on SMO has delivered twice (for surrogacy) and she's been on the list like 5 years or something. She's not sure if she's going to do it again unless someone wants a sibling for the ones she's done already. But, I don't see her leaving the site either. I have no intention of leaving the site either."

Becoming a surrogate

Newcomers discover what it means to be part of SMO by reading discussions and stories and through informative yet at times impatient responses to their posts. Newbies can be criticized for failings that are accidentally revealed by their questions. For example, one newbie posted about her worry of getting pregnant before the embryo transfer because she "cannot always remember to take the birth control pill." Several women told her in no uncertain terms that she "has no business thinking about surrogacy" if she cannot remember taking one pill a day, given that a GS journey involves a rigorous protocol of many different medications for extended periods of time.

Thus begins the "moral career" of a surrogate on SMO.[14] On her way to become a surrogate, and eventually an experienced one acknowledged and respected by others, a newbie has to not only get pregnant and carry a baby for her IPs but also show persistence, openness, good judgment, and independence and strength, and preferably also a sense of humor. She has to deal with medical and legal professionals, make sense of insurance and contract provisions and medicals protocols, and often answer comments by family members, coworkers, her kids' teachers, and even strangers. She then has to manage all this online in the stories she tells and in discussions with others. She not only has to go through the stages of the process but also honor the stages by listening and deferring to women who have gone before her.

This collective understanding affirms the value of accumulated knowledge and more experienced surrogates' position in the SMO hierarchy. At the same time, newcomers are reminded how much work it is to become a serious candidate and eventually a good surrogate. SMO is not simply a gathering place for women interested in surrogacy; rather, it is a forum that helps forge interest into determination and action that is consistent with group expectations and norms. Group norms, according to most surrogates, include the right to criticize but also tolerance, fairness, and equality. When these norms are violated, some surrogates step up to remind everyone that criticism is fine, but meanness is not, not even from experienced old-timers: "Neither you, nor anyone else should be worried about being crucified about ASKING something or answering something. Are there experience police on this board? Good grief. SMO SHOULD be a board for newbies to come and feel safe, NOT a place for crotchety b*tches who 'lash out' at someone."

Nevertheless, threads do attest to the importance of "experience." But what constitutes experience? Discussions reveal that women attain surrogate status by carrying a child for IPs; birth to a viable baby, however, is not a necessary criterion. Going through testing, matching, contract negotiations, embryo transfers or artificial inseminations, and some of pregnancy seem to be sufficient for the surrogate title. This is in keeping with surrogates' insistence that surrogacy is not a commodity transaction, and as much as a healthy baby is the goal, it is not the ultimate measure of a surrogate.

Having done at least some of the journey is transformative: newbies become surrogates. However, they are once in a while reminded of how much they will still have to learn and experience: "what does bother me is the know-it-all attitude of some surrogates when they haven't completed a journey." Surrogates exercise social control on SMO; being acknowledged and approved by more experienced surrogates bestows status more than the simple fact of pregnancy. SMO discussions bear out Goffman's point about the ultimate importance of the organization of social control.[15]

SMO-organized social control works through discussions. SMO-ers often preface their posts by delineating the limits of their experience and thus of the validity of their advice. There is widespread recognition on the boards that it is important to acknowledge where one is in the journey. Pregnant surrogates often introduce posts by saying they are not experienced but offer advice based on their journey so far. This is a good strategy. Unless newly pregnant surrogates position themselves between newbies and experienced surrogates, thereby acknowledging the distance they have yet to travel, they are sooner or later reproached for assuming too much. Some threads directly take up the question of experience: "What do you count as experience? If someone has cycled once are they then given the SMO green light to speak about it? When does someone become not a newbie and 'allowed' to speak up in posts that pertain to things they have done/are doing without others feeling put off by it?"

A three-time surrogate offered a summary: "If you've personally 'been there, done that' then you have that particular experience." As surrogates move from matching and testing to attempts at achieving pregnancy—through artificial insemination in TS and medication and embryo transfer cycles in GS—to pregnancy and birth, they gain experience not only about the legal and medical process but also about the emotions and relationships involved in surrogacy. They also become experienced in effectively discussing and deciding all these issues with fellow surrogates.

Experience, as in other areas of life, comes from accumulated knowledge and practice. For credible claims to experienced status, one completed journey, especially an easy one, may not be quite enough. Credible, and honored, claims are normally based on having experienced difficulties and complications or more than one journey. Experienced surrogates offer "narrative maps" to newcomers; their authority derives from personal involvement, from "having been around" and "through" those domains of life and having accumulated both factual and personal knowledge in the process.[16]

They often feel obliged to respond to newbies, even though they may not always appreciate the questions, as the following quotation indicates: "When we do have a lot of crazies, I tend to stay away from responding to questions from new members . . . , but . . . I would hate for new members to be drawn away for lack of response." Experienced surrogates developed and cultivated a sense of responsibility not only for upholding standards but also for the continued functioning of SMO, whose very existence depended on participation.

Nevertheless, sharp criticism is not uncommon. Some women generated more drama or controversy than others. "SMO-holics" readily recognized the drama potential in posts. "I'm getting out the popcorn," they joked. The most active and vocal women carved out unique roles for themselves, such as storehouses of knowledge of past discussions, peacekeepers when discussions got out of hand, or the voice of reason in emotionally laden threads. They voiced strong opinions and displayed distinctive character traits. Others referenced these traits and roles, thereby demonstrating familiarity and creating personalized conversations.[17]

Women also often referred to past differences of opinion with others. "I cannot believe we are in agreement about this, Connie!" one surrogate teased another with whom she had regularly locked horns. And when Mona announced, "I may be done w/ surrogacy for myself, but I am an SMO addict, and I think I'm gonna stay," she received warm responses. Hedi teased her for staying only for her "boob threads," meaning the threads Hedi started about plastic surgery options. Vivian reminisced about their differences: "I'm so glad you aren't going anywhere. While we tend to disagree, I appreciate your honesty and frankness! It serves as my wake-up call!"

These references were reminders of a shared history and ongoing association in which camaraderie, at least ideally, trumps difference. They expressed appreciation no matter what else may also be true, and focusing on the things that united SMO-ers contributed to a sense of solidarity.[18] Alluding to past events, debates, positions, or others' character traits was also a vehicle for women to display their intimate knowledge of both fellow surrogates and SMO history and thus highlight their insider status.

How to think about the field site

Thinking about SMO as an "opportunity structure"[19] for "temporary interactional enterprises"[20] guided my decision to approach it as my field site. My investigation was informed by grounded theory, with its focus on discovery and building theory from data, and by the Chicago School of sociology, with its emphasis on understanding the actors' viewpoints and the centrality of the interpretive process in order to grasp social interactions and practices. Herbert Blumer's injunction is as valid as ever: "Respect the nature of the empirical world and organize a methodological stance to reflect that respect."[21]

My study of SMO is essentially an ethnographic exploration of this online world of surrogacy. At a time when Internet-based practices increasingly mediate and shape assisted reproduction, my research brings into focus surrogates' own discussions of the issues most salient to them and the ways in which these discussions contribute to women's desire to become surrogates. My work focuses on surrogates' communications not only because they are the most active presence on the boards but also because, contrary to public perception, they play a major role in propagating surrogacy.

Jack Katz pointed out that "the single most common warrant for sociological ethnography is that what is obvious to the subjects has been kept systematically beyond the cognitive reach of the ethnographer's audience."[22] Additionally, "ethnographies have a widely recognized ability to depict communal realities," and on both counts the warrant is to make what is obvious to SMO-ers known to others.[23] The media's focus on surrogates' personality traits and fascination with individual stories notwithstanding, I found "what ethnographers always find: that people act collectively and that what outsiders think of as the product of individual personality is in fact the result of social interaction."[24]

Mine is not a conventional ethnography. I did not attend support group sessions, nor did I observe surrogates in clinics or doctors' offices. Yet my investigation looks "directly at social action by particular social actors in particular social times and places."[25] The social action in my case is online communication and the place is SMO during its decade-long heyday. I observed interactions on SMO message boards by reading discussions and debates among participants (surrogates and some intended mothers) about many surrogacy- and non–surrogacy-related topics for more than ten years.

Christine Hine contended that online ethnographies are "almost but not quite like the real thing."[26] But what is real? Online interactions lack the physical and spatial dimensions typically associated with ethnography, yet they are real to the people who engage in them and should be real to the researcher as well. Hine maintains that "the concept of the field site is brought into question. If culture and community are not self-evidently located in place, then neither is ethnography."[27] I discussed some aspects of the SMO community earlier and will go into more details in later chapters. Here, I only want to briefly take up the issue of place and culture as it relates to my field site.

It is true, as Hooley said, that "no one lives online,"[28] but no one lives in a physical support group, either. Discussions reveal that SMO was the main support site even for those members who attended agency-organized support groups. While agency-organized physical and online support groups are for the duration of the surrogacy process, SMO had a longer lifespan and more continuity for the many members who stay for years, including periods of time between or after surrogacies. SMO is clearly considered a *place* by surrogates; women from different locations and backgrounds come here for information and support. Metaphors testify to the conceptualization of SMO as a place; women talk about "hanging out" there and "not leaving SMO," and they greet surrogates who had taken some time off with "so glad you've come back!"

After some months off the boards, Ellen was happy to "stop by": "haven't been here in a LONG time!! Nice to see some familiar faces." SMO also makes physical meetings possible. Women often ask, "where in X state are you?" or realize they live close by as they read posts on SMO; many offline friendships would not have been possible without SMO mediation. Without SMO, most women would not have known about other surrogates who lived nearby or near the places they traveled to visit clinics. Most importantly, surrogates appreciated, even cherished, the ease with which they were able to be part of this surrogacy world and were proud of its distinctive features. They liked the fact that queries were answered fairly quickly and counted on receiving responses from women who had similar experiences or problems.[29]

The *culture* of SMO is the product of the ongoing process of discursive practices. Unlike in agency-mediated support groups, women create, modify, and maintain the tone, style, and standards of communication, and they exercise social control without institutional guidelines.[30] Both physical and online support groups are entities of changing composition where people come together for periods of time. However, there are more opportunities on SMO for branching out to discuss many other aspects of life unrelated to surrogacy. Time and place are not limiting factors and neither is group composition; women are able to post and respond to posts at their convenience and talk to those interested in the same issues. These varied discussions about private matters generate more connections and camaraderie, draw women closer, and reinforce standards of communication and support.

"Communication is at the core" of the "sociology of culture"; "collective representations . . . exert a strong social force."[31] Collective representations emerge as people make meaning together in specific social settings. SMO is such a setting, and women's multiple discussions weave the complex "webs of significance" that "constitute culture," in this case, the emerging culture of surrogacy.[32] Such webs of significance are of a special character because SMO discussions leave a written record for anyone to find later. Past threads become a repository of knowledge.

Aspirations and desires often resonate differently within these webs of significance than outside of them. For example, critics may see repeat surrogacies as a confirmation of commodification, but surrogates certainly do not. Wanting to do more surrogacy journeys is both a desire to "create families," a much-praised endeavor by women on SMO, and a signaling of commitment to fellow surrogates and intended parents.

The virtual is real

SMO transcends geographical distance, yet it is overwhelmingly a site for US surrogates and intended parents, allowing easy communication among the interested parties. By communicating directly, surrogates and IPs also bring about change in the social organization of assisted reproduction. By talking to one another online about the legal, financial, medical, and emotional aspects of surrogacy, surrogates learn not only what they want to know, they also learn what they *should* want to know. They learn about group practices and expectations, and they learn to participate and thus actively produce and reproduce the online world of SMO. Information and advice in a social setting that is unfamiliar to newcomers "is both about a social world and part of the process through which a social world is produced and sustained."[33]

The exchanges were often strikingly intimate, as women discussed both surrogacy-related and other issues and created "webs of personal relationships in cyberspace."[34] Lisa told me of her own experience:

> I have actually made more friends [here] than I have since I was in school (nearly 20 years). I correspond daily with a lot of them, chat on AIM or Yahoo Messenger and what not. One lady miscarried her own surprise pregnancy and a lot of women pitched in and put forth money and bought her a puppy she really wanted, flew it across the country to her and delivered it to her door. And it wasn't even surrogacy-related. Just pure friendship.

Online communication allows "access and intimacy" that is not transferrable to face-to-face situations.[35] Ava told me that "any problem that I could experience, out of the hundreds of women on there, SOMEONE has experienced the same thing. I can turn there for help on absolutely everything."[36] Women were able to post anytime with relative ease, and someone was likely to respond soon. The expectation that this was indeed the normal course of events is exemplified by a typical query by a surrogate whose post went unanswered for a day: "How come nobody responded? Please, ladies, I see many of you read my post, but here it is again."

Online advice transcends simple transmission of information; it is also a ritual sharing, a choice of and commitment to the online community.[37] Anthony Cohen proposed that "we try to understand 'community' by seeking to capture members' experience of it."[38] Surrogates, especially the more involved members, experience SMO as "socially real" and "consequential."[39] Community is often understood not simply or primarily as a bounded location but as "a quality of holding something in common, as in community of interest . . . a sense of common identity and characteristics."[40] SMO enables a discursive process of common identity formation. The interactional definition of community is especially useful here: "Community is constituted by individual identification of and involvement in a network of particular association."[41] For understanding SMO, it is useful to think about community in terms of communication: "Community is . . . the communicative process of negotiation and production of a commonality of meaning, structure, and culture."[42]

New communication technologies "enabled new strategies through which social actors connect."[43] By interacting, women established connections on SMO that were the source of real, rather than virtual, support; it provided real, rather than virtual, appreciation.[44] "It's just a great community of women supporting women."[45] For example, when Abby posted about a recent ultrasound showing that the fetus stopped growing at seven weeks, forty-three fellow surrogates posted sympathetic messages over a period of three months, and several indicated that they called or talked to her in person.

Surrogates do not typically receive this kind of empathy off the boards; often even their own families do not understand why they are heartbroken over such an early miscarriage when it is someone else's child. Women posted about real joy and real pain and often said that SMO was the only place where they were fully understood. "I wanted to start off by saying that I'm a very private person but know that you ladies are the ONLY ones who would be able to relate to this in my life." Such expressions point to one of the key features of community, namely that "people have something in common with each other."[46]

Surely, having something in common is not a given in any setting, and it does not automatically lead to a sense of community. SMO was the venue where members together formed and developed real and meaningful connections both online and off and thus created the things they had in common and recreated SMO as the place for women who have things in common. Scholars have documented how members of online groups who foster close relationships make

efforts to also meet face-to-face.[47] SMO-ers took every opportunity
to meet in person; they posted about upcoming travel plans to see
who is in the neighborhood. In some instances SMO-ers offered a
room to a fellow surrogate who traveled for embryo transfer. Women
planned offline get-togethers online; for example, a Northern California surrogate invited everyone who could make it to her house
for a summer weekend. At times surrogates sought assistance from
fellow SMO members. One such case was a request for transpor-
tation for the husband of a hospitalized surrogate; several women
volunteered. SMO-ers helped one another in various emergency
situations. For example, one surrogate got violently sick from food
allergies while traveling to meet her IPs. After her IM dropped her
off at the airport, she was too sick to travel and contacted a local
fellow surrogate, who picked her up, took her to the ER, and put her
up for another couple of days while she was recovering. Women also
organized collections for buying presents for fellow surrogates whose
journey ended particularly badly. The online and offline realms
are not strictly separable. Countless posts testify to the importance
of both the on- and offline camaraderie and the shared sense of
identity and purpose despite occasional disagreements, bickering,
or even sharp criticism. SMO members "exercise immediate social
control upon one another" through frequent communications and
develop strong, meaningful, and enduring emotional "technological
ties that bind."[48]

The owner of the site periodically reminded members of the
importance of self-control: "Please, please remember that this is
a public board and we have thousands of people that read it every
day." Some of the less than civil debates shed light on an important
issue: the public nature of the site. Women take it on themselves to
chastise others for breaches of civility. The following is a comment
on an uncivil post:

> When things turn ugly in a surrogacy relationship, I find it extremely
> unprofessional to take sides publicly and post your opinion in a
> public forum. . . . This is a PUBLIC PLACE. Would you act this way,
> face to face, standing in the middle of, let's say, the mall? It's shame-
> ful. Typically, I would handle this privately in PM or email.

The woman whose post was ostracized defended her actions: "I have
EVERY right to say what I am feeling. If someone was spreading lies
to NUMEROUS people about you, I think you would say something
about it to. I am not going to sit back and watch someone spread lies
and hurt others without saying something about it."

Several SMO-ers knew the story and some took sides, but most others maintained that such exchanges were inappropriate: "This stuff needs to stop! SMO is NOT the place for it!" The owner of SMO had the last word: "If you . . . don't like someone, ignore them or take your issues with each other off the boards and do it privately." It is thus made clear that certain communications or styles of interactions are inappropriate, and standards of behavior are upheld. The standards themselves, much like group norms, are revealed mostly only when they are violated.

Surrogates collectively constructed what was public by also delineating what was not. "What we choose to share is up to all of us," as members can privately e-mail one another through their profiles. Choices about what to disclose were shaped by somewhat contradictory considerations, such as surrogates' respect for privacy, their desire for broad support, and their aspiration to be the public voice of surrogacy. They asserted that while protecting participants' privacy is important, it is equally important to post "the good, the bad, and the ugly" so that others, including future readers, may be educated. This orientation to a perceived or potential audience generates an important public dimension. Diane, for example, was concerned that some threads about a surrogate's "absolutely terrifying past" had been removed from the boards. She made a case for the importance of public accountability: "People reference SMO when they are matching to ensure that the people they are talking to aren't crazy or a danger. On one hand, yes, it's 'just' a message board. But on the other hand, SMO has become the backbone of the surrogacy world."

Women affirmed the importance of both honesty and community and of a community based on honesty: "Don't lose your voice," warned Jess, "whether done intentionally or not, silencing voices can be dangerous. Especially in a community such as this." Judging from the numerous personal stories and impassioned debates, women heeded the advice to make their voices heard:

> Each one of us has something unique only we can teach others. Every person we come into contact with throughout life has a lesson to teach us. It's our responsibility to learn those lessons and pass them on. . . . Quite frankly some parts of surrogacy may not be positive but we shouldn't be silenced simply because it may make surrogacy look bad to others. Our honesty may be what helps the next person to not be hurt in the name of surrogacy. Being hurt sucks. It's what we choose to do with that hurt which is important. We can let it eat us away a little at a time or we can take a stand

and try to help others avoid it. One of my biggest lessons has been in choosing my words to get the message across in ways that others will be able to hear.

SMO members usually took their educational role very seriously and saw the boards as the best forum for it.

There are other signs indicating that women regarded SMO as a public space. SMO members typically welcomed former "lurkers" who post about joining SMO. "I'm new here! I've been lurking. . . . I didn't want to pipe up much until I knew I'd be moving forward with surrogacy. I figured I mostly need to read and learn, anyway." Posts by newbies who confessed to lurking often implied deference and admiration for the "ladies": "I'm mostly a lurker too, mainly because I don't know half of what these other ladies know." This "proper deference" elicits warm responses on SMO.[49] Members routinely welcomed lurkers with "Glad you decided to join," "Welcome! Best of luck on your journey!" and "You're in the right place!" This attitude represents an acceptance of lurking behavior as appropriate and an implicit acknowledgement that the space is public.[50] Thus lurking is not a violation of privacy but preparation for surrogacy and SMO membership; it is responsible behavior, not eavesdropping.

There is a further sense in which online discussions are public. Online linguistic behavior, as Davis and Brewer argued, is a hybrid form, combining the characteristics of both written and oral interactions.[51] This kind of communication interactively builds common experience and shared values; it constructs shared worlds. And as Cavanagh and Robinson and Schultz suggest, online linguistic behavior constitutes interaction in Goffman's sense, involving strategic self-presentation and ritualized forms of interaction.[52] When I followed discussions on SMO, I was not observing individuals; rather I was observing interactions that constructed the public online world of surrogacy. Surrogates' online communication interactively built common experience and shared values; it constructed shared worlds.

Once in a while one member let another know that she had private information that she promised to share in e-mails or on the phone, and the recipients often publicly posted about having received the private communication. These public announcements about private communication are interesting, given that women could have simply e-mailed or called one another without letting others know. Posting about private communications advertised the existence of an inner group that shared information and news that others on the boards were not privy to. At the same time, these posts signaled the need for occasional privacy and also willingness to offer help beyond the boards. It also enabled women to get credit on SMO for their help even when it happened beyond the public eye.[53]

Surrogacy beyond SMO

SMO's increasing importance for surrogates was partly due to the increasing heterogeneity of the organizational and regulatory practices of assisted reproduction. The proliferation of agencies, fertility centers, and even law firms specializing in surrogacy has led to increased competition among them. All this seriously eroded the hegemonic position intermediaries used to have at the time of Ragoné's writing.[54] At the time, women interested in surrogacy signed up with one of the very few existing agencies and followed their procedures. Now, women can do online research, compare agencies, and negotiate with them based on information they gleaned.[55] More experienced surrogates also reminded newbies that they do not have to give up all control: "An agency can often honor the requests you mentioned. . . . Many agencies are flexible, just ask :-)."

SMO-ers posted extensively about the pros and cons of the professionals (agencies, clinics, doctors, lawyers) they had worked with. Mattie, for example, was quick to post her negative experience as well as her solution to the situation. "I have nothing good to say [about the agency]. . . . Luckily I was not a newbie that got sucked in. We were matched then we walked away from the agency and continued our journey." Her post generated quite a bit of enthusiasm. "I'm so glad that you are getting the word out and hopefully . . . we can eventually get some regulation and lock up all of these shady agencies and REs [reproductive endocrinologist]!" There are long threads about surrogacy-friendly health care providers by state, with special emphasis on gay-friendly ones.

Surrogates are increasingly able to find IPs with the help of lawyers or independently. More experienced surrogates are more likely to opt for an "indy journey" because they accumulated more knowledge about the process. Many women who use an agency for their first surrogacy think of it as a learning experience: "you learn SO much from letting an agency show you the ropes the first time. It's a great education in surrogacy." Surrogates insist that taking charge of the process is a must: "No matter which route you chose, you

STILL have to do your own research." SMO-ers have formulated a general principle of individual responsibility. "Know what the normal process and steps are and don't skip a single thing, even if an agency says something is unnecessary. Whether you go indy or not, ultimately your journey is your responsibility to get right."

This possibility to gather information and gain knowledge is both liberating and burdensome. The Internet, according to some scholars, is a site "for generating new forms of knowledge, awareness, and agency"[56] and "helping to shatter the professional 'information monopoly,' allowing lay people to understand their situation in detail, compare notes with others, reconstruct knowledge . . . and find support."[57] The Internet, however, also generates new forms of responsibility to do research and find the relevant information and knowledge. Information gathering is guided by both practical and emotional considerations.[58] Surrogates who seek information often also want to hear encouraging outcomes and uplifting stories.

My findings indicate that for surrogates the Internet does reduce inequality and has effectively eliminated the "information monopoly" agencies used to enjoy. Gaining medical and legal knowledge helps to "level the hierarchical relationships" between agency personnel and surrogates and, more recently, between clinics, doctors, and lawyers on the one hand and surrogates on the other.[59] Gathering information from SMO and other Internet sources and comparing notes with many other surrogates enables women to be active, prepared, and well-informed participants in a practice that centrally involves their bodies and their physical, emotional, and financial well-being. SMO-ers thus took on the responsibility to educate themselves and others, and by doing so they also assumed responsibility for presenting surrogacy in a favorable yet realistic light on a public site.

Methods: "let our stories guide you"

Observing online

Online observational techniques are well suited to focusing on linguistic behavior in natural settings, as they occur in the field—in my case on SMO.[60] Online linguistic behavior is a hybrid form, combining the characteristics of both written and oral interactions; this overlap is favorable for exploring the complexity of meaning, offering the benefits of both interpersonal involvement associated with talk and "the elaboration and expansion of thought associated with writing."[61] SMO-ers creatively used emoticons, font, and capitalization to infuse written words with more nuanced emotional expression.

My mostly passive presence on the boards had definite benefits for my research; I was unimportant to the participants.[62] I did not interfere with what women discussed or how they discussed it. I was able to observe the interactional dynamics on SMO without ever setting the agenda. Becker noted that a "volunteered statement" is less likely to reflect the observer's "preoccupations and possible biases" than one that is a response to the observer's actions or questions.[63] He pointed out that "the observer's very question may direct the informant into giving an answer which might never occur to him otherwise.[64] On SMO it is surrogates' own questions and interests that drove discussions; all SMO discussions are "volunteered statements." Women brought their own concerns to the boards, formulated questions, and raised issues—often repeatedly.

Becker also pointed out that no social situation is what it would have been without a social scientist present even if no one knows that the social scientist is a social scientist.[65] This truth about presence is relevant in my cyber–field site. Women knew that increasingly many different people—intended parents, future surrogates, journalists, students, researchers—read their posts. They referenced this readership, whose presence as audience had certainly shaped SMO discussions.

Since I was neither a surrogate nor an intended mother, I did not participate in discussions but made my presence on the boards known as much as was possible. I contacted the owner and explained my research and she gave me permission—not that permission was necessary—to quote from posts as long as I did not reveal anyone's identity and did not "show surrogacy in a bad light."[66]

I posted two requests, explaining my project and asking surrogates to contact me. Overall, thirty-five surrogates responded in e-mail, some only briefly, others in several follow-up e-mails, sometimes prompted by my question "How is your journey going?" I met with one surrogate, Shanna, in person when she came to Los Angeles for her transfer, and we arranged to meet again after the first one failed.[67]

These women's stories and responses corroborated my reading of the online discourses; they used very similar language and articulated ideas, hopes, and experiences akin to what I have seen in SMO posts. I asked women about SMO discussions, and they commented on some controversial threads and well-known debates. I treat these responses not merely as individual stories but as elucidations, confirmations, and sometimes clarifications of the stances I encountered on the message boards.

All but five of the surrogates I corresponded with were employed, mostly in secretarial and support jobs, and all said they were middle class. Four were divorced mothers, the others married with two to four children. There is no comparable demographic information about SMO members. Discussions, however, revealed that most participating surrogates were married and had two to five children. They had regular access to computers and spent time reading, commenting, and advising. Many of the women had impressive legal and medical knowledge. Gestational surrogates compared notes about cysts and high blood pressure to assess if these could be the possible side effects of the hormones they take. Citing statistics and posting links to new medical findings, surrogates passionately debated embryo transfer practices and multifetal pregnancy outcomes. They were proud of being well informed and proud of taking risks, saying that "surrogacy is worth sacrificing for."

In the initial phase of my research, I followed threads about women's dreams and expectations about surrogacy, the matching process, contract negotiations, and their relationship with IPs during pregnancy and after birth. The more I read, the more I realized that in order to get a full picture of the site and the women on it, I needed to read forums I had not considered at first. For example, "Just chit-chat," "In the news," and "Support" contain a mix of surrogacy- and non–surrogacy-related communications. These threads allowed me a glimpse into women's lives through their discussions about children, husbands, in-laws, work, cars, guns, books, and news.[68] One can also glean information from the informal polls SMO-ers initiate about a variety of topics. Reading these threads put surrogacy-related discussions in social context.

From discussions, stories, and polls the following picture emerges. Almost all surrogates are white and mostly between their midtwenties and late thirties. The majority is Christian, yet surrogates are quite strikingly liberal on gay issues. "Spiritual" is also a common self-characterization. A minority does not vaccinate their children at all, and quite a few vaccinate selectively. There are many stay-at-home mothers, but the majority works full time as nurses, teachers, doulas, lab technicians, dispatchers, legal and accounting assistants, paralegals, information technology managers, account managers, office managers, software testers, and massage therapists.[69] Some own small businesses.

Informal income polls reveal that the majority of surrogates who responded had a yearly family income of more than forty thousand dollars, excluding surrogacy compensation. The majority of women who answered poll questions about educational attainment had more than a high school degree. While none of the anonymous polls are statistically rigorous and it is impossible to know what proportion of SMO surrogates responded, the many polls and posts I have read over a decade in which women discuss their lives, as well as women's writing style and their attention to spelling and grammar,[70] indicate lower-middle- to middle-class status, not lower class and financial desperation, as many critics assumed.[71]

I followed thousands of discussions over the years, and certain approaches, styles, and stances were rather consistent while memberships changed and grew.[72] But while I pieced together a qualitatively detailed picture of the interacting group, I know less about individual women. My goal, however, was to capture shared definitions and the range of accounts that emerge from collective debates rather than document individual stories.

The nature of my mostly observer role, as well as my non-ideological interest in surrogacy, offered guarantees against over-involvement, yet I came closest to it when Lisa lost her job after she delivered her second surrogate baby and was unable to find a full-time position. I knew Lisa had chosen to continue working with her second couple even though they were somewhat insensitive at the time of her earlier miscarriage. And I could not really blame the couple for not responding in substance to Lisa's e-mails about her unsuccessful job search. What is the right thing for IPs to do in a situation like this? After all, they were not responsible for supporting or even helping her financially beyond their contractual obligations. They may have feared to express too much ongoing sympathy, worried that it could be interpreted as taking responsibility for Lisa's job loss.

I knew that her IPs were making good on their promise to send her updates and could not be realistically expected to do much else, yet I found their lack of empathy troubling. Even as I understood the delicacy of the situation, I was angry and sympathized with Lisa. Then she told me she needed to move to a cheaper place and asked me to lend her fifteen hundred dollars for the deposit. This provided further insight into the emotional complexity of many surrogacy-related situations and the politics, and economy, of sympathy.

Local knowledge

Logging on to SMO several times a week allowed me to learn to "appreciate local meanings and concerns" and to familiarize myself with "members' explanations and theories"; it also enabled me to see both consensus and change emerge from debates and conversations.[73] Becker pointed out that "the nearer we get to the conditions in which [people] actually attribute meanings to objects and events, the more accurate our description of those meanings will be."[74] Meanings are generated about and attributed to surrogacy-related feelings and events in many settings, but even these externally arrived at meanings are brought to SMO for collective scrutiny, discussion, and often redefinition. And SMO itself is a site for generating and attributing new meanings. Meanings are consequential: people's actions are "based on the understandings of their local social worlds."[75] "Story and meaning" are "the grounds of agency and intentionality."[76] Grounded theory's assumption that "the social world studied through fieldwork is inherently narrative-bound" is literally true for SMO.[77]

SMO exchanges are narratives, some longer and fuller than others. Surrogates communicate about their experiences, which are in many ways a "breach" of the ordinary and as such call for stories.[78] These stories are not simply accounts of individual hardships or victories; they "connect people" and help shape group identity.[79] Stories impute responsibility and "lend themselves to moral evaluations."[80] Narratives do not simply describe events and experiences but "construct and negotiate interpretations," and people "use those interpretive frames to guide future action."[81] SMO narratives help surrogates not only make sense of experience and find solutions to problems but also identify problems and decide what is worth solving.

Reading threads is the best way to understand surrogates' joint efforts at meaning making. These meanings cannot simply be "discovered"; rather, they are the result of the interpretive and analytical work of the researcher.[82] This work begins by taking members' meanings seriously as "naturally occurring situated interactions in which local meanings are created and sustained"[83] and continues with letting "the case define the concept."[84] I follow Becker's call for "developing concepts in a continuous dialogue with empirical data."[85] As Elijah Anderson put it, "The ethnographer should enter the field armed with a certain sociological sophistication, even a theoretical perspective that . . . helps to formulate questions" but "the orienting questions should emerge from the local knowledge the researcher gains from the field setting, not just from his or her intellectual preconceptions."[86]

Such "intellectual preconceptions" are not rare in the scholarship on reproduction. For example, Barbara Katz Rothman contends that "any pregnant woman is the mother of the child she bears" because of the social relationship between the fetus and the gestating woman.[87] Rothman's strong preconception is that "every woman bears her own baby . . . regardless of the source of the sperm, and regardless also of the source of the egg."[88] She further argues that in surrogacy this relationship is discounted; the baby becomes a "commodity, something a woman can produce and sell."[89]

Rothman's method of inquiry is the opposite of mine. Rothman defined the concept of motherhood and concluded that surrogacy represents the case of the commodification of motherhood, while I privilege surrogates' definitions and views of motherhood and of the relationships of surrogacy. To appreciate their positions we need to start with surrogates' "ethnonarratives," which originate in their experience and understanding of the social world and are the "basic building blocks" of ethnographic analysis in the grounded theory tradition.[90] I took my "theoretical clues" from the discussions I read on SMO.[91] As the empirical data show, surrogates and intended mothers see motherhood rooted in intent and desire, rather than genetics or gestation.

This kind of investigation into native definitions takes us closer to understanding the growing practice of surrogacy. The issue at hand is not to decide what motherhood is; rather, it is to understand what the parties to surrogacy hold to be true and how these definitions inform, encourage, or discourage certain practices. The ethnographic approach "discourages reified accounts and too-easy generalizations . . . highlighting agency rather than deterministic outcomes."[92] Surrogates clearly exercise agency in debating and defining the various concepts and practices that constitute surrogacy.

Agency, in Sewell's definition, means being "empowered by access to resources of one kind or another," and SMO is such a resource for its members.[93] Women's actions and decisions are shaped and informed not only by online advice, stories, and discussions but also by the emerging moral consensus on SMO about what it means to be a good surrogate. This is a world I set out to explore and understand. My goal was consistent with the goal of ethnography as Elijah Anderson defined it: "to provide a truthful representation and analysis of the social and cultural world of the subjects."[94]

In some Internet-based projects researchers asked how people used the site and what they thought of being on the site.[95] Sustained reading of SMO posts yields this kind of information in its own rich context.[96] Discussions reveal what is important to the women who engage in them and provides insights into the social and cultural world of its members. Women repeatedly started threads about issues they cared about, and important topics gave rise to heated debates, attracting thousands of "views" and frequently ten times as many responses as most other threads. For example, there could be no mistaking the vital importance of threads about how many embryos to transfer or about termination and selective reduction.

Clarifications and confirmations

Yet, as much as it is informative to know what surrogates discuss on their own initiative, it is important to hear what surrogates say about these discussions if asked directly. So although my project is about the social dynamics of SMO discussions, about how these online communications lead to crystallizations and contested or agreed-upon definitions of the practice, my e-mail correspondence with surrogates provided some additional insights.

Examples of such a confirmation and elaboration are from my correspondence with Angelina and Ava. I asked about a stance I had noticed on SMO, namely, that surrogates seem to think that all intended parents who want a child deserve one. Surrogates carry not only for infertile childless couples but also for people who are past childbearing age, have grown children from a first marriage, or have several young children and wish to add to their family. Extremely few women said they would only carry for a child-less couple. The ones who did were often a bit defensive about it, explaining that they did not want to judge who deserves a child but thought it was "more special" to carry for people who were childless. Some were quick to add that they did not mean that *they* want to be more special, just that the experience would be so for the IPs.

Angelina explained her own thinking: "My reason for wanting to help a couple is because I can't imagine not having my three chil-dren. I would have been just as devastated if I could only have one child because you have that 'dream number' in your mind."[97]Ava wrote, "The mentality of SMO is that everyone has the right to have a child, no matter what. Unless an IP comes forward and they are absolutely, blatantly nuts, the board will support their right to have a child. Anytime one person speaks out against someone's rights to have a child, there will be backlash."[98] At the same time, Ava insisted that she decides for herself. "Sometimes I'll admit my eyes may be opened, or I may feel more compassionate toward a situation than I did before, but I still feel solid on who I will or will not work with."[99]

These exchanges confirmed my understanding of who were considered "deserving IPs" on SMO (pretty much everyone who wanted to have a child) but also directed my attention to the ways in which this general stance played out in individual decision making. Surrogates' decisions about which IPs to choose were compatible with, and did not negate, their nonjudgmental position. It is clear from their stories that individual characteristics and "chemistry" were often more significant than abstract principles. However, stories also indicate that some surrogates, swayed by the notion of deserving IPs, disregard warning signs and match with couples about whom they had misgivings.

Some of my e-mail exchanges with surrogates proved to be informative in ways that I had not anticipated. For example, I commented on how many of the stories I had read on SMO were not good ones and how devastating many surrogates seemed when IPs cut ties or redefined the relationship as business after the baby was born. While several surrogates agreed with and added to my observation at first, they quickly became defensive. I was initially taken aback by this reaction because surrogates so clearly wanted me to be sympathetic rather than simply curious. But as I was "learning the rules of the group" that were "amorphous, and heavily dependent on the situation,"[100] I had come to realize that criticizing IPs could be problematic. Thinking about women's responses further, I recalled the following relevant observation: in SMO discussion, sympathy for surrogates who felt betrayed by their IPs' distancing behavior was increasingly often balanced with "giving IPs the benefit of the doubt." SMO-ers pointed out that IPs were too busy; they needed time to bond with the baby and needed "space" to become a family.

Criticizing IPs was not a simple matter. My position was especially delicate because, being an outsider, I certainly could not know enough either about these specific cases or about the lived experience of a surrogacy relationship; I had not earned the right to criticize IPs. Surrogates were possibly also protective of the good memories of their relationship with their couple. But there was more to it than this. As I came to realize, surrogates did not want me to take their side; rather, they wanted me to be prosurrogacy.

In the context of much media attention to bad stories, any criticism could potentially turn into a critique of surrogacy itself. If IPs could be so unfair or ungrateful, can it still be true that they are "wonderful people who deserve a baby?" Women often reiterate that just because some IPs did not treat their surrogate well it does not mean they will not be great parents; the need to repeat this contention indicates that it is not resolved and may not be resolvable. Criticizing IPs is an uncomfortable reminder of this and potentially calls into question the central purpose of surrogacy, to help "great couples become parents."

Another instance of unanticipated and indirect information had to do with motivations. Even though I never asked, women almost always told me why they became surrogates. They seemed to assume I wanted to know, and I assumed they thought so because everyone else asked them this question. Their answers were not surprising, as answers to "why" questions tend not to be.[101] Women often said they knew someone who had infertility issues or heard some news report about a couple who had, and these stories broke their heart. They told me how much they loved their children and could not imagine life without them and how they were helpful and giving people by nature.

I noticed that surrogates periodically started threads on SMO with titles like "Why did you become a surrogate?" Put in this context, their e-mails revealed a new set of meanings. They told me their stories not so much as an answer to my unasked question but because they liked to tell moral stories about the value of children and family, of helping and giving behavior. These explanations as to why they had decided to become surrogates "passed muster" not only in the eyes of an imagined audience but in their own eyes as well.[102] Such answers to their own questions proved that they were the kind of people they had aspired to be.[103]

Dealing with data

In the beginning stages of my research I extensively read posts on SMO message boards to see what topics women discussed and how they discussed them. After familiarizing myself with the site, I started to keep notes on discussions, outlining the issues and positions women articulated, the way the discussion or debate developed, and whatever else "was going on" and saved links to threads. Increasingly, the sheer amount of data became a problem. Lisa's joking remark that I was "hooked on SMO" was not a joke. My frequent visits did not always yield new data but simply more data. It took me a while to come to terms with this conundrum: the very thing that was so easy about this research—data at my fingertips—

was also a hurdle. Ironically, the ease with which I was able to see "what my surros were up to" made seeing what they were up to in a deeper sense more of a challenge.

I began writing memos, which helped to keep the data more organized and raise more questions about the concepts I was developing. Memo writing enabled me to explore emerging themes, for example the connections between surrogates' characterization of their relationship with IPs and other SMO-ers' reactions to these accounts. I started with broad themes, such as "disappointment with IPs," and as I read and reread my data and sought answers to my questions about it I developed more specific categories.[104] For example, I noticed that disappointed surrogates did not always get sympathetic responses; in fact, some reactions to such posts were quite accusatory. Given that surrogates usually get support when they find themselves in bad situations, I took lack of support to be a negative case that enabled me to make further distinctions. These negative cases helped me to recognize systematic differences between various types of disappointments and prompted me to ask new questions about the stories.

Analyzing the negative cases led me to distinguish cases in which "IPs 'were not there' for surrogate" from cases in which "IPs went back on their promises." Sorting my data in these more specific types of "disappointment" categories enabled me to understand the variations in SMO-ers reactions to different stories. Responses were typically all supportive when IPs did not keep promises. Not keeping promises is a clear violation of an agreement and is uniformly condemned. IPs' lack of support, their "not being there for the surrogate," however, was understood as a subjective evaluation of the situation that had to do with expectations rather than agreements. Although women often empathized with disappointed fellow surrogates, they also criticized those who seemed to have unreasonable expectations and came across as too needy or not strong enough to deal with less than ideal situations, especially as surrogates increasingly defined the "good surrogate" as informed, strong, loving, and independent.

Memo writing enabled me to make further distinctions. For example, memo writing focused my attention on the difference between members' reactions to complaints by surrogates who at the same time affirmed the value of surrogacy ("venting") and their responses to pure complaints ("whining"). Vents by surrogates who expressed determination after experiencing disappointment were met with practically unanimous praise and encouragement, while whining got much more mixed reactions.

Most women labeled their own complaints-plus-resolve posts as "vents" and others agreed, often saying "it's OK to vent, Honey!" However, no one called her own complaint "whining"—others did. Vents showed resolve, generosity, and strength in the face of hardship, whining, on the other hand, meant self-pitying complaints. The former was in keeping with the surrogacy ideal; the latter clearly was not. Those who approximated the collective ideal were rewarded with sympathy and praise, and those who were too sorry for themselves were often chastised. Comparing reactions to stories was a good way to sort my data and more systematically discover patterns of variation, and thus patterns of significance.

Together, the *patterns* of discussions—that is, the way some topics persist, others disappear, and yet others intensify over time—and the *modes* of discussions—that is, sympathy, criticism, praise, or censure and their combinations and proportions—reveal how online communications shape meanings. Surrogates produce and sustain collective understandings and crystallizations about this new practice without intermediaries, and, at times, against pre-established hierarchies of knowledge. "I absolutely appreciate you coming here to tell your story . . . this is exactly how we all learn to make surrogacy work!!! "Through validation, praise, censure, and criticism surrogates on SMO collectively worked out not only the definition of "the good surrogate" but also the ethos of surrogacy.

Although women assume they have somewhat similar experiences and views to other members when they join SMO, they still have to build bridges between "members from so many different areas and walks of life," especially in a new social practice in which so little can be taken for granted and shared understandings cannot be counted on. They need to create and sustain common ground in order to understand others and be understood by them. It is not meaningful to seek and receive advice and support unless people on the boards share some basic understandings of what the goals, behaviors, and emotions of surrogacy are. Surrogates produce and sustain these collective understandings and crystallizations about this new practice without intermediaries, expert opinions, or pre-established hierarchies of knowledge. "I absolutely appreciate you coming here to tell your story . . . this is exactly how we all learn to make surrogacy work!!!"

The strange and the familiar

One of the basic paradigms of anthropology and sociological ethnography is that the field is foreign. Even as anthropologists and ethnographers increasingly explore settings close to home, "making the familiar strange" is a prerequisite for "making the strange familiar." SMO was far from familiar to me; it was foreign land, and I had to learn its language. It was through written words that I have come to understand these women; both IMs who struggled with infertility and surrogates who wanted to help them. My only common ground with them was my love for my own children; neither infertility nor assisted practices had been part of my own life.[105]

Trying to understand social practices through immersion in written communications poses obvious limitations for my study. I do not know what women do when they meet with IPs for the first time or during contract negotiations or doctor's appointments; I only know what they write about these events. However, there are a few points I want to make about the connections between discussions, practices, and how they matter for my project.

First, when surrogates talk about practices among themselves, they compare notes and ask for advice and information. They want response, guidance, and reassurance; misrepresenting their case would be counterproductive given that they look for useful and meaningful answers.

Second, they tell their stories knowing that many IPs, including their own, and several surrogates they know personally are, or are likely to be, reading on the message board. In some instances, surrogates and IPs posted their own version of events, and several others, who had firsthand knowledge of what had happened, also chimed in. Experienced surrogates take pride in their ability to catch inconsistencies between past and current posts. Contentious and contested exchanges testify to the possible challenges any post faces, whether it bends facts or not; every story has at least two sides, and the various participants impose a check on one other.

Third, even though the previous two points are important for understanding the validity of my data, my project was not designed to evaluate individual practices or probe into individual stories but to understand these online interactions and how they inform and shape collective definitions.

I am careful not to make assumptions or claims about practices I have no firsthand information about. I cannot directly see practices, only the ways in which issues are brought up and presented, the ways in which they persist or disappear from SMO. I see how positions get defined and how reactions change, reflecting changing expectations about various aspects of surrogacy, such as the contract, the number of fetuses surrogates are willing to carry, and the relationship with their couple, just to name a few.

Leaving the site

I did not decide how long to stay on SMO when I started this project. It took me a while to understand the reasoning, the references, and the interactions and to work out my methodology. I did not foresee and appreciate the difficulties for the future when I found myself almost drowning in data. Yet staying on the site for this long had the—at the time unforeseen—advantage of witnessing change in a number of different areas as I will discuss in the following chapters.

Even though I knew I had more than enough data when I began writing this book, I could not resist periodically checking SMO to see what was going on.[106] My leaving the site, on the whole, was surprisingly well timed. I noticed slow times, and SMO-ers did, too, a few years ago, but as it turned out, these times were not simply slow but the beginning of an exodus.[107] People still read the site for information, IPs and surrogates still match independently on it, and there are still some discussions. But SMO is no longer "where the action is"; Facebook groups have replaced or at least supplemented SMO in many respects.

The accumulation of information and crystallization of expertise—medical, legal, relational, and emotional—transformed SMO into a repository of knowledge for those who want to read and research. Thus, now women can seek smaller and more congenial groups for support without having to rely on such groups for information.[108] While some Facebook groups may be less contentious, occasional nostalgic posts on the boards bemoan the loss of SMO sisterhood. This book, then, documents the time when SMO's importance and influence was on the rise and the years when SMO-ers proudly called the site the "backbone of the surrogacy world."

Notes

1. New members go through a moderation period. After the owner approves new members (after about thirty posts or when she gets to this task), they have more privileges and can post directly. However, the owner may close contentious threads or ban members who violate rules.

2. January 2013. Just before this, the hosting company upgraded the message boards, leaving the basic organization of the site unchanged. However, many past threads had been deleted (the owner explained that she had to considerably "prune" older threads to make the upgrade possible), and the membership increased considerably after the upgrade.

3. "Announcements" contain information and announcements to members. "General" contains fourteen subforums, such as surrogacy, egg donation, surrogacy news in the media, gestational surrogacy, traditional surrogacy, parents via surrogacy, two somewhat new expert forums for medical and legal issues, respectively (in which a doctor and a lawyer answer questions, often with significant delays), support, pregnancy related, parenting related, and warnings to the surrogacy community. "Our Journeys" contain sixteen subforums, from the "just starting out" and contract and insurance issues to the stages of pregnancy (first, second, third trimester), birth stories, and postpartum and breastfeeding discussions. "International" has few postings in Australian, Canadian, and UK surrogacy subforums. "Miscellaneous" contains twelve subforums from "just chitchat" to surveys, recipes, uplifting stories, world events, get-togethers, etc.

4. I use surrogates' own terms; these terms help us understand the ways in which they create, structure, and understand this online world. I put their terms in quotation marks the first time I use them. However, because quotation marks become both tiresome and a distancing device when used repeatedly, I use these terms without them in subsequent mentions. In my quoted passages from surrogates' discussions, I only corrected spelling and punctuation errors that interfere with easy understanding. I did not correct syntax or intentional misspellings that were meant to indicate sarcasm or criticism.

5. Members are able to interact through their "profiles" not displayed on the public site. Only approved members (those who had gone through the mediation period) are able to select the private e-mailing option.

6. Information about location shows that surrogates are dispersed all over the United States although many live in California, which no doubt has to do with surrogacy legislation. See Susan Markens, *Surrogate Motherhood and the Politics of Reproduction* (Berkeley: University of California Press, 2007).

7. So-called cycling groups, i.e., gestational surrogates whose embryo transfer cycles are around the same time, often form exclusive Facebook groups, where they discuss issues among themselves. These groups are "invitation only" and are usually composed of women who already know or have some connection to one another.

8. While surrogates use the term "former intended mother" in its abbreviated form (FIM), they do not typically use it for IMs who are active on the boards. Surrogates use numerical differentiation, such as "my first IPs." "Former" indicates closure, while "first" and "second" simply indicate chronological order.

9. Howard S. Becker, *Doing Things Together* (Evanston, IL: Northwestern University Press, 1986), Becker made it clear that he did not mean only face-to-face interactions; see Howard S. Becker, *Outsiders* (The Free Press, New York, NY, 1963), 182.
10. "Journey" is the most commonly used name for surrogacy; I will discuss this in detail in Chapter 2. On the subject of doing only one surrogacy, Hal Levine found that lack of support was a decisive factor in surrogates' decision not to do further surrogacies. Hal B. Levine, "Gestational Surrogacy: Nature and Culture in Kinship," *Ethnology* 42 (2003): 173–85.
11. All my quotations are from SMO, unless otherwise indicated.
12. Lori Kendall, "Recontextualizing Cyberspace: Methodological Considerations for On-line Research," in *Doing Internet Research: Critical Issues and Methods for Examining the Net*, ed. Steve Jones (Thousand Oaks, CA: Sage, 1999), 58.
13. Surrogates use terms such as "betrayed," disappointed," or "let down" when intended parents break their promises, are distant, or cut ties. To be a better person means to be a proud surrogate in the face of disappointment and while acknowledging the hurt, move on without too much bitterness.
14. Erving Goffman, "The Moral Career of the Mental Patient," *Psychiatry: Journal for the Study of Interpersonal Processes* 22, no. 2 (1959): 123–42.
15. Erving Goffman, *The Presentation of Self in Everyday Life* (New York: Doubleday, 1959).
16. Melvin Pollner and Jill Stein, "Narrative Mapping of Social Worlds: The Voice of Experience in Alcoholics Anonymous," *Symbolic Interaction* 19, no. 3 (1996): 204, 207.
17. This is similar to how regulars at an electronic lesbian café "use . . . knowledge [of others' lives and characteristics] to personalize conversation" online. Shelley Correll, "The Ethnography of an Electronic Bar: The Lesbian Café." *Journal of Contemporary Ethnography* 24, no. 3 (1995): 290.
18. SMO-ers interact online, which makes it easier for them not to reveal or discuss political views than it is for people who have to physically coordinate their activities. As Courtney Bender suggested, leaving ideological differences aside facilitates group solidarity (Courtney Bender, *Heaven's Kitchen: Living Religion at God's Love We Deliver* [Chicago: University of Chicago Press, 2003]). However, in the early 2000s there were some heated debates on SMO about the Iraq War; many women were enthusiastically for it, suggesting, "We need to blow the place up and be done with it." Some others were antiwar, insisting that it is "not up to the US to decide the fate of the people of another country." Military wives said they supported the troops and the president. Some others pointed out the political complexities and that it was a mistake to invade, given that it was not Iraqis

who attacked the World Trade Center on 9/11. Things flared up again when the Abu Ghraib abuse cases got publicity. In these discussions many participants expressed their love and support for Bush, which made others irate. Another topic was homelessness, which stirred up some passions, prompting several women to tell their own stories of hardship and struggle, spelling out the key difference, i.e., that they are willing to work while homeless people are not. These debates left surrogates with some bitterness toward one another. "This is why I don't discuss politics with people," wrote a disgruntled surrogate. At the time of the Sandy Hook school shooting, most women resisted the temptation to respond to posts that addressed the issue of gun control, opting instead to agree that loss of life is tragic, especially when it is children's lives. A few corresponded about the advantages of home schooling. To be sure, it is impossible to know how much women care about certain political issues or whether they simply decided not to discuss them. However, the earlier heated debates did seem to have left women with a lesson that it is best to avoid divisive issues, especially if they have nothing to do with surrogacy.

19. Gary A. Fine, "The Sociology of the Local: Action and Its Publics," *Sociological Theory* 28, no. 4 (2010): 356.
20. Erving Goffman, *Interaction Ritual: Essays on Face-to-Face Behavior* (New York: Pantheon Books, 1967), 2. Interactions on SMO are occasioned by questions and stories, and even the longest threads are temporary as new questions and stories, new responses and reactions arise.
21. Herbert Blumer, *Symbolic Interactionism: Perspective and Method* (Englewood Cliffs, NJ: Prentice-Hall, 1969), 60.
22. Jack Katz, "Ethnography's Warrants," *Sociological Methods and Research* 25, no. 4 (1997): 393.
23. Ibid., 415.
24. Ibid., 400–401.
25. Andrew Abbott, "Of Time and Space: The Contemporary Relevance of the Chicago School," *Social Forces* 75, no. 4 (1997): 1169.
26. Christine Hine, *Virtual Ethnography* (Thousand Oaks, CA: Sage, 2000), 10.
27. Ibid., 64.
28. Tristram Hooley, Jane Wellens, and John Marriott, *What Is Online Research? Using the Internet for Social Science Research* (London: Bloomsbury Academic, 2012), 77.
29. Sharf also found that members of the breast cancer support e-mail list she studied appreciated quick responses, and she learned about the varied experiences and expertise of others. The support e-mail list included many more people than any physical support group could have, offering advice and support around the clock. Barbara F. Sharf, "Communicating Breast Cancer On-line: Support and Empowerment on the Internet," *Women and Health* 26, no. 1 (1997): 65–84.

30. Troll detection, i.e., the identification of people whose posts purposely stir up trouble, is one way to monitor the site. Troll-suspicious posts are considered fair prey and treated with disrespect: "Sounds like a lying drama-seeking troll that knew enough to sound real for about 30 seconds. All it took was a couple people asking reasonable questions to blow it for her." Surrogates are very quick to identify inconsistencies, improbable details, or uninformed descriptions in a post, and, invariably, someone investigates and quickly posts the results. Then they make fun of the perceived attempt to deceive them: "I love it when people come here and think they're soooo much smarter than the rest of us. Especially people who don't use proper English, appropriate grammar and good spelling. Yep, just a bunch of dumb a$$ serrogants here, we'll NEVER figure out that she's posting as both a Surro and an IM." When they believe they have exposed a troublemaker, SMO-ers proudly declare, "Trolling FAIL." However, almost all of the troll detections I have followed turned out to be false alarms; troll-suspicious women often came back to explain that their questions or stories were genuine, but they were away for some days and thus unable to respond. They almost invariably swore never to post again on such a hostile board. These instances prompted some SMO-ers to reiterate the value of a less judgmental approach.
31. Nina Eliasoph and Paul Lichterman, "Culture in Interaction 1," *American Journal of Sociology* 108, no. 4 (2003): 735, 736.
32. Clifford Geertz, *Interpretation of Cultures* (New York: Basic Books, 1973), 5.
33. Pollner and Stein, "Narrative Mapping," 204.
34. Howard Rheingold, *The Virtual Community: Homesteading on the Electronic Frontier* (Cambridge, MA: MIT Press, 2000), xx.
35. James T. Costigan, "Introduction: Forests, Trees, and Internet Research," in *Doing Internet Research: Critical Issues and Methods for Examining the Net,* ed. Steven G. Jones (Thousand Oaks, CA: Sage, 1999), xxii.
36. Ava, e-mail communication, 26 April 2010.
37. Steve Jones, "Studying the Net: Intricacies and Issues," in *Doing Internet Research: Critical Issues and Methods for Examining the Net* (Thousand Oaks, CA: Sage, 1999), 15.
38. Anthony Cohen, *The Symbolic Construction of Community* (London: Tavistock, 1985), 19–20.
39. Richard Jenkins, *Social Identity* (New York: Routledge, 1996), 111.
40. Raymond Williams, *Keywords: A Vocabulary of Culture and Society* (New York: Oxford University Press, 1983), 75.
41. Mary Virnoche and Gary Marx, "'Only Connect'—EM Forster in an Age of Electronic Communication: Computer-Mediated Association and Community Networks," *Sociological Inquiry* 67 (1997): 86.
42. Jan Fernback, "There Is a There There: Notes Toward a Definition of Cybercommunity," in *Doing Internet Research: Critical Issues and*

Methods for Examining the Net, ed. Steve Jones (Thousand Oaks, CA: Sage, 1999), 205.

43. Karen A. Cerulo, "Reframing Sociological Concepts for a Brave New (Virtual?) World," *Sociological Inquiry* 67, no. 1 (1997): 52.
44. Cerulo (ibid.) makes a similar point about CompuServe e-communications. Victoria Pitts ("Illness and Internet Empowerment: Writing and Reading Breast Cancer in Cyberspace," *Health* 8, no. 1 [2004]: 33–59), Patricia Radin ("'To Me, It's My Life': Medical Communication, Trust, and Activism in Cyberspace," *Social Science & Medicine* 62, no. 3 [2006]: 591–601) and Clive Seale ("Gender Accommodation in Online Cancer Support Groups," *Health* 10, no. 3 [2006]: 345–60) observed powerful expressions of support on websites for breast cancer patients.
45. Ava, e-mail communication, 26 April 2010.
46. Cohen, *Symbolic Construction,* 12; Williams, *Keywords,* 75.
47. E.g., Amy Bruckman, "Identity Workshop: Emergent Social and Psychological Phenomena in Text-Based Virtual Reality," unpublished manuscript, MIT Media Laboratory, 1992, http://www.academia.edu/2888780/Identity_Workshop; Lori Kendal, "Recontextualizing Cyberspace: Methodological Considerations for On-line Research," in *Doing Internet Research;* Sherry Turkle, "Cyberspace and Identity," *Contemporary Sociology* 28, no. 6 (1999): 643–48.
48. Karen A. Cerulo, Janet M. Ruane, and M. Chayko, "Technological Ties That Bind: Media-Generated Primary Groups," *Communication Research* 19, no. 1 (1992): 109, 113.
49. Shelley Correll, "The Ethnography of an Electronic Bar: The Lesbian Café," *Journal of Contemporary Ethnography* 24, no. 3 (1995): 293.
50. Allison Cavanagh, "Behavior in Public? Ethics in Online Ethnography," *Cybersociology Magazine: Research Methodology* 6 (1999), accessed 28 November 2009, http://www.cybersociology.com/files/6_2_ethicsinonlineethnog.html.
51. Boyd H. Davis and Jeutonne P. Brewer, *Electronic Discourse: Linguistic Individuals in Virtual Space* (New York: State University of New York Press, 1997).
52. Cavanagh, "Behavior in Public?"; Laura Robinson and Jeremy Schultz, "New Avenues for Sociological Inquiry: Evolving Forms of Ethnographic Practice," *Sociology* 43, no. 4 (2009): 685–98.
53. I am grateful to Alice Goffman for calling my attention to a more complex reading of these public announcements of private communications.
54. Heléna Ragoné, *Surrogate Motherhood: Conceptions in the Heart* (Boulder, CO: Westview, 1994).
55. Numerous threads provide information about the kinds of freedom agencies allow surrogates (setting fees, contract provisions, etc.). In 2008 I conducted telephone interviews with the directors of three large California-based agencies (all three asked not be identified), who

told me that potential surrogates often come with clear ideas as to what they wanted in their contract; they all thought this was the result of Internet-based information.

56. Pitts, "Illness and Internet Empowerment," 34.

57. Radin, "To Me, It's My Life," 600.

58. Ibid.; see also Michael Hardey, "Doctor in the House: The Internet as a Source of Lay Health Knowledge and the Challenge to Expertise," *Sociology of Health and Illness* 21 (1999): 820–35.

59. Pitts, "Illness and Internet Empowerment," 43.

60. Chris Mann and Fiona Stewart, *Internet Communication and Qualitative Research: A Handbook for Researching Online* (Thousand Oaks, CA: Sage, 2000), 85.

61. Davis and Brewer, *Electronic Discourse;* Mann and Stewart, *Internet Communication,* 189.

62. Howard S. Becker, *Sociological Work* (New Brunswick, NJ: Transaction Publishers, 1970).

63. Ibid., 30.

64. Ibid.

65. Howard S. Becker, "The Epistemology of Qualitative Research," in *Ethnography and Human Development: Context and Meaning in Social Inquiry,* ed. Richard Jessor, Anne Colby, and Richard A. Shweder (Chicago: University of Chicago Press, 1996).

66. I am mindful of issues of privacy and do not include URL citations; I also changed all the names and do not take posts out of context.

67. The second time one of her intended fathers (she matched with a gay couple) came to the transfer from New York and was in her hotel room, visiting. Soon after I arrived another intended father came with three bags full of takeout food. These intended fathers met through their surrogates who became friends on SMO. Shanna's friend's IFs lived in Los Angeles and took this opportunity to meet Shanna and one of her IFs. We sat around and had a picnic on the king-size bed, where Shanna was resting after her transfer, and gossiped about SMO characters. This transfer failed, too, and the couple decided to work with a different surrogate. The next time I heard about them was from a front-page *New York Times* article after their second surrogate had delivered their baby. Shanna went on to have a baby for a heterosexual couple, which ended in heartbreak for her; her IM barely kept in touch during the pregnancy and severed ties after the baby was born.

68. E.g., discussions about parenting emphasize communication with but also setting limits for children. Discussions of husbands and porn tend to conclude that "men will be men."

69. Countless discussions about contractual specification of reimbursement for lost wages and the use of sick leave for surrogacy also indicate the prevalence of employment.

70. Bad spelling and poor writing are mercilessly ridiculed on SMO.

71. E.g., Gena Corea, *The Mother Machine: Reproductive Technology from Artificial Insemination to Artificial Wombs* (New York: Harper & Row, 1985); Sara A. Ketchum, "Selling Babies and Selling Bodies," in *Feminist Perspectives in Medical Ethics,* ed. H. Bequaert Holmes and L.M. Purdy (Bloomington: Indiana University Press, 1992), 264–94.

72. SMO had around 800 members in 2002 and around 32,000 in 2014; numbers include both surrogates and IPs.

73. Robert M. Emerson, Rachel I. Fretz, and Linda L. Shaw, *Writing Ethnographic Fieldnotes* (Chicago: University of Chicago Press, 1995), 109, 124.

74. Howard S. Becker, *Tricks of the Trade* (Chicago: University of Chicago Press, 1998), 14.

75. Emerson, Fretz, and Shaw, *Writing Ethnographic Fieldnotes,* 139.

76. Sherry B. Ortner, "Introduction," *Representations* 59 (1997): 11.

77. Iddo Tavory and Stefan Timmermans, "Two Cases of Ethnography: Grounded Theory and the Extended Case Method," *Ethnography* 10, no. 3 (2009): 257.

78. Jerome Bruner, "The Narrative Construction of Reality," *Critical Inquiry* 18, no. 1 (1991): 11; Jerome Bruner, *Making Stories: Law, Literature, Life* (Cambridge, MA: Harvard University Press, 2003); Arthur W. Frank, *Letting Stories Breathe: A Socio-Narratology* (Chicago: University of Chicago Press, 2010).

79. Frank, *Letting Stories Breathe,* 60.

80. Charles Tilly, *Why? What Happens When People Give Reasons . . . and Why* (Princeton, NJ: Princeton University Press, 2006), 16.

81. Charyl Mattingly, *Healing Dramas and Clinical Plots: The Narrative Structure of Experience* (Cambridge: Cambridge University Press, 1998), 9.

82. Emerson, Fretz, and Shaw, *Writing Ethnographic Fieldnotes,* 108.

83. Ibid., 140.

84. Becker, *Tricks of the Trade,* 123.

85. Ibid., 109.

86. Elijah Anderson, "The Ideologically Driven Critique," *American Journal of Sociology* 107, no. 6 (2002): 1536.

87. Barbara Katz Rothman, *Recreating Motherhood* (New York: WW Norton, 1989), 243.

88. Ibid.

89. Ibid., 236.

90. Tavory and Timmermans, "Two Cases of Ethnography," 253.

91. Ibid., 244.

92. Robert M. Emerson, "Ethnography, Interaction, and Ordinary Trouble," *Ethnography* 10, no. 4 (2009): 536.

93. William H. Sewell, Jr., "The Concept(s) of Culture," in *Beyond the Cultural Turn. New Directions in the Study of Society and Culture,* ed. V.E. Bonnell and L. Hunt (Berkeley: University of California Press, 1999), 10.

94. Anderson, "Ideologically Driven Critique," 1537.

95. E.g., Correll, "Ethnography of an Electronic Bar"; Clare Madge and Henrietta O'Connor, "Parenting Gone Wired: Empowerment of New Mothers on the Internet?" *Social & Cultural Geography* 7, no. 2 (2006): 199–220.

96. Posts are text, and as Cavanagh points out in "Behavior in Public," "We tend to see text as autonomous, produced in isolation" and thus assign authorship to it. But in many contexts, and SMO is one such context, text is produced cooperatively as part of ongoing talk; they reflect interactions rather than authorship.

97. Angelina, e-mail communication, 30 March 2006.

98. Ava, e-mail communication, 5 April 2010.

99. Ibid.

100. Elijah Anderson, "Jelly's Place: An Ethnographic Memoir," *Symbolic Interaction* 26, no. 2 (2003): 232.

101. Jack Katz, "From How to Why: On Luminous Description and Causal Inference in Ethnography (Part I)," *Ethnography* 2, no. 4 (2001): 443–73.

102. Ibid., 445.

103. Goffman, *Presentation of Self.*

104. Kathy Charmaz, "Grounded Theory," in *Contemporary Field Research: Perspectives and Formulations,* ed. R.M. Emerson, 2nd ed. (Prospect Heights, IL: Waveland, 2001).

105. I was surprised to find this to be powerful common ground. Lisa's e-mails, containing inspirational poems about motherhood, made me tear up even as I intellectually objected to their sentimental content. Over time, I learned to relax and accept my tears while holding on to my objections. It was interesting that peer reviewers often assumed that I was familiar with the site for reasons other than academic and asked me to "clarify" my interest in it.

106. A small proportion of my data is from more recent discussions.

107. A surrogate returning to SMO posted the following in August 2014: "Is it just me or has anyone else noticed SMO seems less active lately. It seems like it's been like that ever since I've been back (I had twins in late Oct and stopped checking . . .)." Others saw this as well: "I've noticed it too. It was always a hopping place back a few years ago." Some commented on the advantages: "It seems to get busier when the crazies come out and then quiets down when they leave. We are in a crazies lull right now." Soon, another explanation was offered: "Most people are on FB groups now. You don't have to sugar coat and blow smoke up everyone's butt." The reply was quick: "Yeah, except that they gang up on people, then someone ends up getting hurt, deleted and friendships end. That's real nice. I like it here where we have to be civil." On the whole, however, Facebook groups are "where the party went," as a long-timer said in 2014, although several surrogates wish for the return of the "good old times."

108. Elizabeth Ziff confirmed that this was indeed the case, and I am grateful to her for the following elaboration: "I think your sense about the way SMO is used nowadays is correct. Even though from what I understand these women aren't actively using SMO the way they used to, it is still one of the first resources they reference when newcomers post messages on the FB page asking for information. Really, not a day goes by that I don't see a link to SMO and I would guess it has to be due to the rich resources there. A handful of surros that I have spoken with did use SMO regularly and have transitioned to FB because they feel that SMO has become 'trashy' or 'catty'" (private communication).

Chapter 2

JOURNEY

Surrogates most often talk about the purposeful endeavor to create a child as a journey of shared love. They have a varied cast of companions other than intended parents—husbands, fetuses, and fellow SMO-ers—on their journey. This chapter is about the ways in which surrogates fashion these relationships through stories, debates, and discussions and about the role of the love rhetoric in establishing common ground for the participants. I follow the narrative chronology of the journey.

First, I will chronicle discussions about husbands, family members, and friends and the roles they play as surrogates prepare for the journey. Then I will discuss surrogates' relationship with intended parents as they embark on the journey. Third, I demonstrate the ways in which surrogates see, negotiate, and debate their relationship with the fetus they carry. Fourth, I discuss surrogates' expectations of and relationship with their intended parents during the pregnancy and following the birth. I also document their reactions to "loss" during the journey. Fifth, I take up the ways in which surrogates collectively rethink surrogacy and reaffirm their relationship to fellow SMO-ers at the end of the journey.

"I had to explain to him . . . why I felt WE should do surrogacy"

Husbands

Most surrogates are married women and thus husbands are the first to hear about their plans to carry for others. "I want and NEED to be a surrogate. I know I was made to do this," posted Caitlin, who was trying to persuade her husband for two years, asking how others did this. Experienced surrogates advised her—and other newbies with similar problems—to research surrogacy together with her husband and discuss all the issues as candidly as possible. Some women volunteered their husband: "if he would like open communication from another hubby I am sure mine would speak to him," wrote Bella. She said she felt the way Caitlin did and even though her husband was hesitant at first, talking it over helped: "I NEED and FEEL [surrogacy] is something I was meant to do. He listened and we went from there."

Another surrogate wrote "Give it time, it's normal for a DH [darling husband] to be shocked at the beginning. But if you keep mentioning it and he sees this is something that you really want to do he'll support you." Taking years to convince a husband is not that unusual. "It took my DH almost 2 years before he realized that if I was still talking about it, it must be very important to me." For many women it took quite a bit longer: "It took me 7 years to convince DH to let me do one surrogacy," wrote Bella. "I'm sure he has valid reasons and concerns. The best you can do is try to give him info, and wait it out," advised Naomi, who waited for five years.

A few women suggested that while explaining everything is essential, highlighting the monetary benefit may be a good strategy. "This really is something I would love to do, for so many different reasons. I think the financial benefit is what's going to have to be the convincing factor for him, unfortunately! But, whatever it takes—as you have said I most definitely will need his support." A few women who went against their husband's wishes offered their stories as cautionary tales to emphasize that no one should embark on surrogacy unless her husband is supportive: "He was GREAT for my first TS [traditional surrogacy]. Was ok with my 2nd. But not very helpful and was very distant. With my last TS, it broke our marriage. He was not for it and I did it anyway," Stephanie wrote. She then concluded: "The love of surrogacy is temporary, the love of a partner should be forever."

Ragoné argued that surrogacy enabled women to gain more domestic power and freedom from their husbands.[1] I found that surrogates on SMO emphasized their husband's contribution and expressed gratitude. The possible bias of these accounts notwithstanding—women may not want to acknowledge marital frictions, even to themselves—it is significant to note the complete absence of the distancing behavior Ragoné theorized about. Women discuss marital decision making in various threads and overwhelmingly describe their marriage as a "partnership" in which they make "joint decisions." Annabel's post represents a typical formulation: "We work together on big decisions and always come to an agreement together. . . . when we're at an impasse we work it out. If it is something that is very important to him I may relent but he reciprocates."

The language surrogates use to discuss their husbands is not the language of "empowerment" but of companionship and shared goals. Neither is there evidence that surrogates "use the monetary compensation they receive as a means by which to procure their husbands' support for their decision."[2], Money does figure in domestic decision making, but women do not buy their husband's support, just as they do not make independent decisions about surrogacy. Surrogates' first advice is to impress the seriousness of one's interest in pursuing surrogacy on the ambivalent husband. Even women who thought the "financial benefit" would be the "convincing factor" to get their husband on board viewed money as a "carrot" rather than payment or a bribe to secure his support. The only exception I read was Beth's boyfriend's attempt:

> He's saying I should give him money to compensate him for the time he's going to put into the surrogacy!! He said that because he has to get STD tests, be flown (Notice I said flown . . . everything is paid for!) to another state and he has to undergo a psych eval . . . he should be compensated. I was FUMING. I said "Ok, ——, So, how much would you like to be compensated for SUPPORTING ME through something?" He tried to say that's not what he meant. Yeah. Right.

"I'd write him a check for five bucks and tell him to shove it where the sun doesn't shine" was the first response. Others were equally outraged: "Wow. That's all I can think to say right now. Wow. But, no my DH doesn't expect to be paid for ME being a surrogate. Even though we are in this as a family, and my family does benefit, it isn't something he EXPECTS. Wow." Fellow surrogates' responses highlight the SMO consensus that expecting compensation for support and cooperation is not appropriate in an intimate relationship.

By all accounts, money usually did not even come up at first: "At first my dh was unsure. . . . He was right there with me, doing research, reading, learning. As all things in our marriage it was a joint decision." Monica addressed her husband's concerns after she realized he did not fully understand surrogacy and concluded: "Being a surrogate was important to me, but my relationship with him trumps it. I would never dream of trying to talk him into it."

It is important for surrogates that their dream is embraced: "My husband and I went back and forth on my becoming a surro, but in the long run he agreed because it was so important to me. And he did not feel that he should be the one stopping me from fulfilling my dreams."

Betty was looking for advice on how to best convince her husband, who was not happy about a second surrogacy. The "empowerment" approach is noticeably missing from her account: "I know that if I make up my mind and I say, "This is what I want," he'll be on board because it's what I want. But I'd like to address his concerns and know that he's okay with it, not just going through the motions because it's what I want." "My husband is always on board if I'm doing another surrogacy because we are a team . . . and he is on board because he knows it's something I like doing," wrote Lynn.

Reasons for husbands' resistance to subsequent journeys are complex and can only be understood, as I argued before, in the context of companionate marriage:

> i was still wanting to do another surrogacy. . . . But dh voiced a lot of concerns. He didn't want our family to go through what we previously had (bad bad journey). . . . i realized that it hurt him too. That his heart was hurt from it as well. . . . as the carriers we forget how deeply it can affect our spouses. How it breaks their heart to hold our hands and be basically powerless. . . . Finally i realized that he sacrificed a few things while i was a surrogate so that i could pursue that dream of helping a family. Now . . . it's about making a decision for us as a family unit . . . for now it's about US and getting us to a point where he is happy in his career, our kids are set up for life and we love the life we are living.

Natalie similarly took into account her husband's concerns and also retired from surrogacy:

> My husband does not want me to do another journey. . . . I could "convince" him but I don't want to. He was so amazing with everything . . . I don't think I could ever completely give up on having another journey, but for now I am satisfied and so is he. . . . I want to respect his wishes and God forbid something happen, I would never forgive myself for pushing him.

To assert one's independence without regard to the husband's concerns was suggested only as a joke, as a comic reversal of the consensus. Both the childish humor and the disclaimer at the end of the following response signal the shared understanding that no responsible surrogate would ever hold this view: "guess what hubs? im gonna do another surrogacy. put that in ur juice box and suck it. . . . i am completely kidding. i would never recommend anyone to pursue surrogacy if they did not have the support of those closest to them."

Relatives

"Those closest," however, mean mostly husbands.[3] Disapproval from other family members is often treated as an indication of deeper problems with the relationship. "My husband is my major support, if he said no, then I wouldn't. I have no relationship with my mother and her opinion doesn't matter to me." "My family is FULL of headcases and I honestly could care less if I have their support or not," wrote Lydia. Mary summed up her position: "My mother never understood me; why would I expect her to understand me now?" Parents' opposition is not an impediment even when it is understood as well meaning: "My parents have repeatedly stated their objections to surrogacy. I respect their opinions but I am an adult . . . and make my own decisions. I do not like being at odds with them over this, but surrogacy was something I felt drawn to." Another surrogate appreciated her parents' concerns but was equally unyielding:

> My parents were very upset when I told them I was going to be a surrogate . . . to the point of calling me crying, begging me to not do it and offering to pay me whatever amount I would be receiving (which they could afford) if I would not go through with it. . . . Their hearts were in the right place. . . . I appreciated their concern and offer and had this been about money, I would have taken them up on it ~ but it wasn't."

Mothers-in-law are usually dismissed even more summarily. Surrogates often reference long-standing animosity as the reason for the disagreement: "My MIL always thought I was not good enough for her son, and now she can really do me a favor and shut up!" Similarly, "Out of my WHOLEEEEEEEEEEEEEEEE family, it's only my Mother In Law that gives me any sign of disapproval. But on the other hand, she has not liked me since DAY 1!!!! I will continue to be involved in the surrogacy world with or without her!!!" Kim and her husband similarly disregarded family opposition: "My MIL is very against me doing another journey. . . . Her concerns . . . are selfish ones . . . so I really don't care! We are not telling her this time." Other in-laws are usually dismissed in similar ways:

my SIL and BIL . . . They just don't understand why I would do something like this. . . . after thinking about all of this for a few days, I've gotten back to not caring what they think. . . . It made me angry that nobody even wanted to know how I was doing. . . . When I get angry, I feel less vulnerable and much stronger. Screw em.

Sympathetic responses poured forth: "That is how all of my family get togethers are!!! I am like this dirty secret, that if it isn't mentioned, it might go away!! You said it right . . . Screw em!!!!" A number of enthusiastic replies echoed these sentiments. Lilly proposed the following solution for organizing SMO support: "Someone will have to start a screw 'em site!! I'll start a screw 'em thread."

Parents', sisters', and friends' opposition and criticism may be painful but I have never seen it mentioned as a real deterrent. Women often encourage one another to "not mind" pressure from family members: "it is your life, not theirs." Friends' disapproval is frequently discounted as are the friends who disapprove: "she cannot be a true friend if she is not willing to be supportive."

Women periodically discuss their children's attitudes and remarks or ask advice about how to explain or broach the subject so that the kids would be on board. One surrogate started a poll, asking others whether they would consider surrogacy if their children opposed it. The majority of respondents said that as much as it was important to talk to their children about surrogacy, it would be wrong to "cave in" to their wishes. The numerous threads on this topic emphasize the importance of explaining to one's children that surrogacy means helping people become "mommies and daddies."

Many women find that it helps to introduce their children to the IPs and encourage a closer bond so that the children will know who the baby's parents are from the beginning. However, women also advise caution, drawing lessons both from SMO stories and their own experience; bonding with IPs who in the end may cut ties could hurt the surrogate's children. Many surrogates live too far from their IPs for this to be an issue. But ultimately women agree that decisions about surrogacy have to be made by the surrogate and her husband, including how to explain it to children: "You and your husband are the only adults in the house," Mina reminded everyone.

Other than by husbands, not being understood in surrogacy is often taken as proof of the rightness of one's choice, a choice coming from the innermost feelings of the self and thus not decipherable to outsiders. In surrogacy, as in love, "people who have not experienced [it] just don't understand." Kara asserted that "as long as I know what I am doing is right in my heart . . . that's all I care about."[4] For Joy, "a few negatives didn't mean a whole lot to me . . . cause in my heart it was right for us."[5] "Go with your heart on this and good luck," advised Jenny. The heart symbolizes emotions as well as identity.[6] The love rhetoric frames surrogacy as a choice women make because of who they are: empathetic and giving people. Surrogates' emphasis on "the heart" is consistent with the Western cultural understanding that defines love against calculation.[7]

"May you find your perfect match"

Chemistry

Once husbands are on board, surrogates look for intended parents to carry for, which, as we saw from Lisa's example in the Introduction, is not always easy. Excited well-wishers often end their posts with "May you find your perfect match soon." When they find IPs, most surrogates happily announce it on SMO. Countless excited posts about matching with IPs describe feelings of "chemistry" (or even "love at first sight") and the conviction that the relationship was meant to be. These accounts parallel some of the key defining elements of love narratives: "clicking" with and choosing a unique other, sometimes in defiance of the outside world.[8] Marianne followed SMO advice to "listen to her heart" and wait for "the perfect couple" and was happy to report that she found them: "It was just like you all said, when you know you just know."

The language of love is ubiquitous in surrogates' description of their first meeting with the couple. "I fell in love with them the first time we met," Melissa remembers. Rene "was introduced to only one couple and that is where I stopped I loved them from the start." "I LOOOOOOOOOOOOOVE my IPs! We have just recently matched but I already feel SO close to them and am so incredibly excited to be on this journey with them!" This framing of surrogacy is consistent with the understanding of procreation as an act of love in US culture.[9] But journey is a complex metaphor; it evokes space, time, purpose, and the stages of the progress one goes through.[10]

A journey covers distance between distinctive points in space and time, and one can have companions along the way. The etymology of the word goes back to the twelfth century, lending this new practice, surrogacy, the patina of age. Campbell's classic description of the hero's journey proved to be hugely influential for popular psychology and self-help literature, adding a "New Age spice" to the mix.[11] The journey metaphor is also often used for life and love, both commonly associated with surrogacy; "surrogacy is a journey" gains additional resonance because of these linked meanings. Calling surrogacy a "journey of shared love" conjures up images of an intimate joint endeavor that profoundly transforms the participants. Ragoné was the first to explore surrogates' expectations of a lifelong friendship with their couple; agency-organized counseling and support services reinforced the notion that surrogacy is "an ultimate act of love."[12] Surrogates in Roberts's study emphasized "how close they felt" to their couple.[13]

When surrogates invoke their love for the couple, or the couple's love for them, they are highlighting the moral, private, emotional, and unique nature of the relationship, elevating it above the contractual arrangement yet distinguishing it from family relatedness. Surrogates nurture the fetus as the intended parents' "unborn child"; their love for it affirms the bond with their couple. Some women directly compare surrogacy to dating. "I just instantly felt like they were the 'ones'. Sort of like when you're dating . . . and you realize . . . hey . . . I think I'm going to marry this guy! It's the same feeling I think . . . YES . . . there is a perfect match! Just like in a relationship." Jennifer seconded: "When people ask me about the beginning process I often tell them it is like online dating. LOL There is nothing else to really compare it to. . . . The first IPs I talked to I loved."

Numerous threads discuss the role of what surrogates most often call "gut feelings" in the matching process:

> Matching is definitely like dating! Although nerves can set in and make us more anxious, PLEASE trust your instincts about this. If you feel like something is not right, trust yourself. Talk to them and see what kind of response you get. There are way too many surros that don't trust themselves and end up in relationships that they aren't happy in.

An intended mother echoed this understanding, responding to a question about how long it ideally takes for IPs to commit to a surrogate:

> I absolutely think it is about intuition, relationship and chemistry! It can go lightning fast, or snail pace slow and still be perfect. We met three possible SMs before finding our 'true fit'! And the funny thing is, when it is something this serious and personal and so life changing it ends up being like when you met your true love! . . . So don't be scared to move quick on this if . . . your heart says "go for it"!

But it is not always easy to find the "true fit." In a long thread about the reasons surrogates reject IPs after the initial correspondence, several women listed "bad grammar" and "careless writing" as reasons. "I hate to say it, but I didn't even respond to a few e-mails I got because of the horrible grammar/spelling/punctuation. Not just one or two words, I mean the WHOLE THING," confessed a surrogate. "Wutz rong wyth thet?" responded another jokingly. I asked Ava, with whom I corresponded for a while, what she thought of this:

> I feel that you are making a first impression with your emails and if you don't take the time to use proper grammar and spelling, it shows you may not necessarily respect your audience enough to spell some words right. . . . It certainly wouldn't be my biggest reason for telling someone no, although if it were really bad, it could be one smaller detail that leads to a "no".[14]

Her response highlighted the importance surrogates attach to respect and was consistent with the many threads I had read in which respect or a lack thereof was discussed directly. Ava's response was all the more informative because she offered it as her own interpretation of the meaning of careless writing rather than as an answer to a direct question about respect in which she would not have had much choice but to affirm its importance.

Surrogates enthusiastically post about long telephone conversations and e-mail exchanges with their IPs, in the course of which they talk about "just about everything." Self-revelation has been the primary symbol of intimacy since the nineteenth century among middle-class Americans.[15] Women emphasize that good communication, sincerity, and trust are essential. Getting to know one another is the best way to build a good relationship, and experienced members warn newbies not to "jump into" surrogacy. Yet surrogates agree that in many ways a match is a "leap of faith." Over the years an increasing number of threads have discussed the potential of deception and how hard it is to really know how journeys will turn out.

Even though surrogates underline the importance of getting to know IPs and developing a trusting relationship with them, "gut feelings" have a privileged role. "We must have talked on the phone for hours. Right then I knew this was meant to be."[16] Elly Teman reports that Israeli surrogates and intended mothers use the vocabulary of rightness and destiny, of intuitive connection with one another.[17] She argues that through the language of "intuitive knowledge" the parties naturalize and decommodify surrogacy. I found similar narratives of "meant to be" closeness in US surrogates' accounts. The following is a good example of the elusive yet powerful sense of connectedness: "The IM and I have such a connection, we're like sisters. . . . It's really hard to explain, really. I just have this feeling."[18]

This kind of connection is impossible to fully account for because it is not a rational appreciation of the other's attributes that draws us close.[19] The following exchange on the message boards enthusiastically affirmed intuitive knowledge: "Don't ya love it when you just 'click' with your IPs?" "OMG YES! It is like the best feeling ever. It feels like we have known each other for years." When surrogates describe the meeting as "clicking," the match as "meant to be," and their IPs as the "right couple," they narratively situate the interaction in the intimate sphere, where baby making belongs. They enthusiastically report when their husband "hit it off" with the intended father [IF]; this feels like two families coming together as friends. Intuitive knowledge also alleviates possible doubts about the IPs' "real intentions," which are, in the last analysis, impossible to know. SMO-ers point out that some "people will say whatever it is we want to hear to get what they want."

Surrogates would often say that not just their particular match but their whole engagement in surrogacy was meant to be. When women encounter difficulties they often express doubt about whether they had been "meant to be" surrogates. "I have been looking for the right IPs for me. . . . I was losing faith . . . and I started to wonder if this is meant to be or not. Until now . . . isn't it just miraculous when all of a sudden a GREAT couple falls out of the sky?" "I decided that if I didn't feel a connection right away, it wasn't meant to be," explained another woman. "I truly believe with all of my heart and soul that this was one of the reasons I was put on this earth."

Framing surrogacy as a calling shifts the focus from specific intended parents, singular matches, and particularistic emotional attachments to a more abstract and universalistic purpose to help others as the context for "making dreams come true." The conviction that one was called helps women overcome difficulties and disappointments during pregnancy and after birth, while belonging to the SMO community helps to construct, solidify, and sustain this conviction.

SMO-ers often explain their actions by referencing "natural" feminine traits such as compassion, helpfulness, and a propensity for self-sacrifice. The concept of calling satisfyingly unites the different elements that constitute the meaning of surrogacy. To find one's calling means to discover some deep affinity with a course of action and to make a choice that feels right; it combines emotions and competence, agency and destiny. It also asserts the private and nonnegotiable aspect of one's choice; as many surrogates say, "I don't care what others think as long as I know in my heart that I am doing what I was meant to do." This general view of others' opinion is reflected in some siggys: "Don't worry about what people think; they don't do it very often."

But certainty is not that easy to come by. "I dream someday of the perfect journey, is there such a thing?? . . . Why do we do this??? No amount of money makes up for the lost time and stress we put ourselves and our families through." Many surrogates have tried to answer this question. Their explanations range from "because we have a heart of gold" to the more playful "we're all nuts." Lisa, an independent, no-nonsense person with a great sense of humor chose the latter. But most women talk about their reasons in a more serious, even spiritual vein:

> It is something that is in your heart and a calling that you feel you were meant to do . . . it "truly" is a calling. That is why when so many will say that they can't imagine being able to do this and hand a baby over to someone else, I say that is because it isn't "your calling." You have to truly have this calling and passion in your heart to complete this.[20]

There were about four times as many positive as negative responses to the question "Were you called to do this?" in an informal SMO poll, including responses like "I was meant to be a surrogate." Amanda's account is fairly typical of this stance:

> I also feel led to do this, it feels natural to me almost like I have been here and done this before even though it's my first time. . . . I dream about it, a little girl that's meant for someone else and I'm so proud and happy, because I've just helped someone's dream and desire for a child become reality.

Emotions and rationality

To be sure, people use love metaphors in a variety of ways, often while engaging in economic transactions. People "fall in love" with houses, cars, and dresses, which they then proceed to buy. Surrogates, however, use love metaphors in relation to people. When surrogates use the language of love on sites that are read by intended parents, this is not simply a statement about feelings; rather, it is an invitation to and an initiation of a reciprocal relationship.[21] In a letter to her couple she posted on SMO, Marianne also emphasized love:

> Over the last 7 months whilst I've been nurturing this precious little bundle of yours, I've been extra careful. . . . What we have done together has given me so much joy and happiness. . . . The reason that I do care for him is simply because he is yours. . . . Made with love between the 4 of us.

Surrogates, therefore, face an interesting dilemma, partly of their own making. Having framed the surrogate experience as an emotional journey, they run the risk of appearing volatile and irrational. Thus, they balance the emotional and intimate understanding of surrogacy with insistence on contractual obligations, responsibility, competence, and trustworthiness. Yet emphasizing contractual rationality risks appearing cold and calculating, and surrogates navigate away from its impersonal and materialistic connotations. Because there is no language to precisely convey the duality of emotional warmth and trustworthy professionalism, women often alternate between the language of love and that of work. "Some people may not agree with the term 'job,' because as surrogates we don't want to be thought of as employees," wrote Millie, "however, in the broad sense of it, we are. It is our 'job' to carry the child/ren, follow doctors' orders, and abide by our contract."

Becca did indeed disagree with the term. "Surrogacy is definitely not a job. I don't think anyone could pay me enough to carry their baby if I really didn't have the heart to do it. . . .You know that in your heart you really don't think surrogacy is a job. I hope you find a great couple . . . that really will love you." Millie's structural metaphor—surrogacy is a job—"induced similarities" between surrogacy and employment, such as responsibility and obligation, but metaphors provide only a "partial understanding of one kind of experience in terms of another kind of experience."[22] While Millie focused on the similarities, the job metaphor oriented Becca to a key element of difference: that surrogacy, unlike employment, is not simply a market transaction. According to Becca, employees sell their labor power, but surrogates don't sell reproductive services; it takes more than money and the incentive has to come from within.

When Paula asked whether others consider themselves the IPs' employee and surrogacy a job, most respondents did not, although a few found technical similarities between surrogacy and independent contracting. Stacy, like several others, focused on the relationship with her IPs to answer the question:

I am certainly not an employee. It's a mutual project with the parties having different rewards in the end, but a friendship that hopefully will last. If I was an employee, they would be able to decide how and why I should do things. Now we discuss, we agree, or not agree, but ultimately I am in charge of my own body . . . even though I would go to great lengths to do things that are agreeable to my IFs. Therefore, not an employee, but a partner. Fellow surrogates agreed that in the best-case scenario, it is a partnership.

Robin used the word "job" as a synonym for "task": "I knew what my 'job' was. . . . I provided a safe, warm environment for a child." But this is no ordinary job, as Lena was quick to point out, and like Becca, she focused on the meaning of job as employment for money. "Surrogacy is not an 'easy' job. You don't get into it to 'get rich' or to 'make a few bucks.' It's something that's done with every ounce of your heart, soul and life." Women typically reject the market connotations of job as employment, pointing out that any important job entails responsibilities, and that their emotional involvement reinforces their sense of duty to "do a good job." "Just as it is my 'job' to be a good mother, it is also my 'job' to be a good surrogate."[23]

Liana highlighted the difference between two definitions of job, one as "duty," understood as an internalized sense of responsibility, obligation, and purpose, and the other as "employment," defined as following the rules that are the condition of payment:

I originally took the viewpoint that it would technically be a job. Not just any job, but one where I could feel like I was really making a difference in the world. However, . . . I quickly became a service to be bargained for. They did not treat me as though I would do my "job" and give 110%, they felt I needed "incentive" (more comp at the end). This really hurt me. . . . In my mind, it is more of a "duty" rather than a "job." It is something that once I sign my contract, I pledge to create the healthiest environment for their child that I can. . . . You do your job, because it is what you were meant to do.

Discussions show that surrogates display their devotion and caring through strict compliance with contractual obligations and doctors' orders, but compliance is not an indication that they think of surrogacy as a business relationship. Discussions also show that the choices of concepts and metaphors are consequential; they paint a picture that informs and shapes the collective conceptualization of surrogacy.

Samantha, for example, used "trust," "heart," and "work" in one sentence to capture her "perfect" surrogacy experience: "I found an IM who totally trusted me with all her heart and since then I've NEVER regretted my decision to work with them!!!" Tessa's diary also testifies to the "creative importation of meaning" from one realm of experience to another; she used market metaphors to express intimacy and connectedness.[24] After meeting her IPs the first time she asked the intended father "if I should take myself off the market. He laughed and said I could put a big 'SOLD' sign on my belly cause I was definitely off the market! I really liked him then!" When seven-month pregnant Tessa had her second bleeding episode and was hospitalized, she was lonely and scared. "I certainly do not regret any part of my decision to become a surrogate. But I have to admit it was pretty difficult for me that night. I was miles away from my own children . . . and all for a child that's not mine." But as is clear from her narrative, she did it for her couple: "Now I'm truly doing this to bring my dear friends a son."[25]

"It's not my baby"

Fetal personhood and nurturing the "baby"

Although SMO discussions use the words "embryo," "fetus," and "baby" somewhat loosely, "baby" represents a belief about the beginnings of life, and this belief has been debated, challenged, and affirmed on the message boards. The announcement, "we transferred 2 8-cell embabies!!!" is a practical equation of fertilized ova with babies. Many women do not understand how anyone can think otherwise. "To me the terms 'embryo' & 'fetus' are simply other terms that refer to stages of development of a child, just like 'infant' & 'toddler'. A fetus and infant both need a mother or 'host'— another human being to survive."

Early pregnancy detection and monitoring, especially home pregnancy tests and ultrasound technology, contribute to the social construction of the "personhood of the wished-for child."[26] Medical practice and discourse informs public understandings and classifications of pregnancy and fetal development. Recent changes in medical language increasingly differentiate between the pregnant woman and the fetus she carries and also blur the distinction between fetus in utero and baby ex utero.[27] Experimental medical procedures treat the fetus as the patient, who is then often assigned agency and personality.[28] "Fetal medicine is the logical extension of pediatric care to the unborn patient," is the definition offered on the website of a fetal care center.[29]

Differentiation between the pregnant woman and the fetus notwithstanding, if there is one human bond that is widely considered to be natural, it is the attachment between a woman and the child she carries. However, social scientists are weary of natural explanations and instead point out that pregnancy is most of all a social relationship between a woman and her baby.[30] Because of the centrality of this relationship, bonding with the fetus one carries is considered normal. Barbara Katz Rothman insists that "every woman bears her *own* baby."[31] The long months of intimate connection between the woman and the fetus, the unique nurturing relationship that is pregnancy makes "our babies ours."[32]

According to Lauritzen, the "activities of nurturing a child," the caring activity that gestation involves, is constitutive of parenthood; therefore, the surrogate mother is "unquestionably a parent to the child."[33] Although these arguments about the centrality of the mother-child bond steer clear of biogenetic essentialism and naturalistic explanations, they are rooted in assumptions about the "natural characteristics" of women and mothers and thus naturalize social relations.[34]

The claim that pregnancy implies motherhood is formulated as a description but in fact functions as an "incorrigible proposition"—one that is immune to discrediting since it is held to be true no matter what the empirical evidence may be.[35] Thus, when surrogates claim not to have maternal feelings, critics often chalk this up to repressed emotions or false consciousness. But such incorrigible propositions do not help us understand surrogates' experience precisely because they posit attachment as an unquestioned given. Such propositions prescribe "what you are to *say*—it tells you *how to describe*" certain things in the world rather than find out how these things actually are.[36] Empirical evidence suggests that maternal feelings are contingent rather than "normal" emotions.[37]

If we take gestation to be a social relationship, we cannot divorce it from the understandings and meanings people attach to it. According to scholarship on maternal attachment, the process of bonding is facilitated if the pregnancy is planned, confirmed, and accepted and also if the fetus is accepted as a separate individual.[38] Interestingly, these factors work against surrogates' attachment. Arguably, the very conditions for maternal bonding are the conditions for surrogates to establish distance between themselves and the fetus they carry.

What women think about their relationship to the fetus is not simply the outcome of the "nurturing relationship"; in fact, what women think about this nurturing depends to a large degree on the relational context in which it takes place. Nurturance is not a neutral concept; it evokes not simply nourishment or care that guarantees biological as well as social survival but also a set of relationships, attitudes, and priorities that are formulated in the context of a market economy. Nurturing means cooperative rather than competitive behavior, the type of love that is unconditional and enduring, an emotion governed by morality rather than contract.[39]

Surrogates nurture the fetus in ways that are biologically identical to other pregnant women, but they do so in the context of a contractual arrangement, within which, and also *against* which, they uphold the morality of altruism and sacrifice. They nurture the fetus because they had contractually agreed to do so, but at the same time they insist that doing so is an act that transcends market calculations, therefore a gift to the couple. In the context of an evolving relationship with their IPs, surrogates' nurturing relationship is a triangular one; they demonstrate their cooperation with and love for their couple by nurturing "their" fetus. By gestating and thus nurturing the fetus, they are building as well as affirming their social relationship to the couple while also upholding the contractual nexus. Surrogates navigate their relationship to the fetus in the context of their relationship with the intended parents. They often say it is the IPs' pregnancy they are carrying. Surrogates' thoughts and views on relatedness are also more varied and complex than the simple rejection of motherhood, as I will discuss below.[40]

Genetics versus care

All gestational (GS) and almost all traditional (TS) surrogates emphasize that the child they carry is not theirs and they are not bonded with it. "I am pregnant with my 3rd Surro Baby and all I feel is a sense of obligation to them (to be healthy, etc.), but no maternal feelings at all" is a familiar statement on SMO. Gestational surrogates refer to intent—their own to help IPs, and IPs' to be parents—as well as the lack of genetic relatedness as the basis of these feelings. Genetic relatedness—or lack thereof—is not overly emphasized because many IPs use or end up using donated gametes.

Shirley's post exemplifies this understanding: "Surrogacy revolves around intent. A surrogate mother intentionally gets pregnant with and carries a child for someone else. The father of my current IM's future children is a sperm donor. If things don't work out, and she chooses to move on to an egg donor, she will still be the child's mother in my eyes." Many other surrogates concurred. Dotty, for example, "didn't/don't care about the donated eggs/sperm/or even embryos. . . . If it is to help my IPs create the family they are longing for, I am all for it."

Traditional surrogates have more varied narratives. Quite frequently, traditional surrogates describe the relationship as "only biology" or "only DNA." Fran, a two-time TS, advised a newbie who was trying to decide between GS and TS: "we are all the same, doing the same thing, just going about it differently." Kayla, a three-time surrogate summed up the difference between genetic relatedness and parenthood the following way: "My children are mine because of the relationship I've built with them over time. I really don't think that contributing some DNA makes someone 'mine.' Parenting makes a parent . . . not biology." Parenthood and motherhood are somewhat moving targets even though intent is central in assisted reproduction. Rene Almeling documented that egg donors all disclaim motherhood, identifying gestation and sometimes adding the social relationship of parenting as the hallmark of motherhood.[41] Surrogates, on the other hand, unequivocally draw the boundary at parenting—gestation does not make mothers.

The following example illuminates the widely shared definition that neither gestation nor genetics are as essential as desire in determining parenthood. In an answer to Mara's query whether to accept her gestational surrogate's offer to be their traditional surrogate (i.e., "use her own egg") after several failed transfers, Jennifer, a GS, advised her to seriously consider her emotional readiness for the TS situation: "The baby would be the product of your husband + your surrogate. Not to insult your intelligence—I know you already know that." But women on the boards know otherwise. "I don't think I've ever disagreed more with any post I've ever read on SMO. The baby is a result of a mother and father who planned and loved and created their child through a woman who donated something she no longer was using." The outrage was unanimous: surrogates and IMs found Jennifer's post "offensive and insulting."

Women agreed that children are conceived in the "hearts of their parents" and that the "child was hers [IM's] even before conception." "Both of our surrogates saw themselves as egg donors and surrogates wrapped up in one package and it really was that simple,"[42] wrote an IM, conceding that not everyone sees it this way but that those women have no business doing traditional surrogacy. A traditional surrogate offered her perspective: "This was their child that I was carrying, and felt so lucky to be able to give her [the baby] a piece of myself so she could have a body and make it to them." Mara thanked everyone for the advice and firmly embraced the consensus about who the mother is: "I would love to have been genetically connected to OUR baby, but that is not God's plan." In Mara's account, genetic connection to one's child is as much a matter of desire as having a child is; however, neither relatedness nor having a child can be taken for granted.

Another revealing example is when surrogates were mocking a discussion on a different website, quoting one post in particular: "You'd have to be inhumane to not intensely bond with a child you were carrying, even if it wasn't your own." SMO-ers were highly amused by this. "Thank you for the laugh," wrote Monica, adding little red rolling-in-laughter heads. "What an idiot that woman is. She sounds super jealous like she was turned down [by IPs]," wrote Cindy. Discussions reveal that surrogates (and intended mothers) have very different views about the basis of parenthood and the nature of bonding than do critics of surrogacy.

Mimi, who switched to TS after two GS pregnancies, asserted that "my TS wasn't any more difficult than my GS. It's all a frame of mind." Some traditional surrogates, however, believe that it is more than a "frame of mind": "I cannot and will not deny the biological link. I AM his biomom, you can't say otherwise. But I am not his mom. . . . I feel I am detached, I guess?" Prioritizing the social relationship over biogenetic relatedness, Emma asserted, "We are biologically related, that does not make us family." Intention and choice play a key role in these conceptualizations. "Of course M. was always intended to be D.'s daughter, not mine, so I definitely don't think of myself as her mother—biomom or surromom, of course, but not MOM." Dorothy summarized the lesson from SMO posts: "from my reading here, it seems the vast majority of TS do not view their TS babies like they view their own children."

However, there are some traditional surrogates who say that their surrogate babies are their children and describe the relationship as "extended family." Rather than seeing such formulations as simply acknowledgements of motherhood, we need to notice the distancing as well; one's children are usually part of one's *nuclear* family. "Extended family" thus serves the purpose of differentiating between one's own nuclear family and the IPs':

> My surrobabes are my children and i never want to hide that fact
> from them or anyone else. . . . i am their birth mother. Not their
> mom. I love them dearly, but in a different way than i do with my
> own children. Yes, i consider them family . . . extended family. I feel
> the same way about them as you do with any extended family. I love
> them, would do anything for them. I love their parents too and feel
> the same way about them.

This example notwithstanding, "birth mother" is rarely used.
Most surrogates reject this term for surrogacy, emphasizing effort
and planning and that they "did not just get pregnant." SMO-ers
emphasize the distinction between surrogacy and adoption: "if a
child knows . . . that she was created for . . . her parents to have
and raise a loving family . . . that their TS cared enough about them
to help them in such a special way . . . it is not the same as having
an *oops* and deciding you don't want to keep the baby and giving
it up." Intended mothers also object to this term, as the following
example shows: "I consider our surro to be their biomom (not birthmom, . . . to me, birthmom refers to an unplanned pregnancy and
an adoptive placement)." Surrogacy is not simply unlike adoption,
it is the opposite of adoption, women on SMO insist.

The basic premise on SMO is that neither biogenetic relatedness
nor gestation implies "being a mom." All SMO surrogates insist that
the child always *belongs* to the IPs: "we are all carrying someone
else's CHILD! . . . you are carrying the child for someone else therefore that child IS THEIRS! No amount of biology can change this."
Surrogates' metaphors underline the central tenet of surrogacy: that
the fetus-baby belongs to the intended parents. "I'm the babysitter,"
"I'm only the incubator," or "I'm the oven" suggest that surrogates
are an important, but last stage in the process of making a baby;
they will "keep it warm and safe" or "bake" it. This imagery emphasizes that the baby is independent of the surrogate and only needs a
little more "warmth" or "care" before it is ready to be handed over
to its parents, to whom it belongs because of their dream and desire
to become parents.

IPs' desire to have and surrogates' desire to give them a baby is
the main unifying feature of surrogacy: "I don't see a difference
between GS and TS when you are talking about surrogacy and the
TRUE intentions of it!" Surrogates' definition of relatedness cru-
cially hinges on volition: "this child would have never existed if
it hadn't been for the love and desire of the IPs." Focusing on the
intended parents' desire collapses the difference between gestational and traditional surrogacy.

Women on SMO are in complete agreement that desire and love make parents and that surrogate babies were first conceived in the IPs' hearts. The actual conception is often presented as a matter of making some minor adjustments: "What if they started the process fully intent on using their own eggs and/or sperm and found out they needed a donor? I don't think most couples would want to scrap everything when they are getting closer." This post exemplifies the logic as well as the promise of reproductive technology. It illuminates the process by which having one's genetic child with the "help" of a surrogate can easily turn into having a baby with the "help" of donors and a surrogate while holding on to the notion of it being the same baby, the wished-for child of the intended parents.[43]

A surrogate dissented only in principle, not in practice. "Well, I'm the odd one out, b/c I prefer to work with the couple's bio embryos. That said, my first surrogacy, there were donated sperm and . . . I was OK with it . . . (so it really depends)." On the whole, the few surrogates who were less comfortable with donor gametes emphasized that children have a right to know their "origins" and that anonymous donors do not provide "roots." This emphasis on genetic individuality as the basis of personhood and family continuity is consistent with the "geneticization" of identity that Sarah Franklin documented.[44]

However, this genetic origin of roots is logically at odds with the assertion that desire rather than genetics is the basis of parenthood, and loving care makes families, not genetic ties. IPs are often careful not to emphasize genetics too much, possibly because of the uncertainty whether they will be "needing" donor gametes. David Schneider argued that both intentionality—or will—and genetic relatedness are constitutive elements of Euro-American kinship; people are related either by law or by "blood." This conceptualization leaves some room for foregrounding one type of relationship or the other without violating our understanding of what kinship is.[45]

Strathern argued that new assisted technologies emphasize "voluntarism and preference" and reproduce choice; the child is the embodiment of its parents' desire to have a child.[46] Voluntarism and preference are already major components of middle-class nuclear families and family planning in the United States. Relationships with kin are often framed as choice; even as relatedness is a given, relationships are not. Couples decide whether and when to have children, how many, and how far apart. In the middle-class imagery of the nuclear family, the child completes the family of its parents, but its connection to other members of its extended family are less taken-for-granted.[47] In many important ways, assisted reproductive practices tap into contemporary middle-class thinking about childbearing and relatedness.

Studies of surrogacy in other countries shed comparative light on the issues. Israeli surrogates emphasize genetic relatedness between fetus and the commissioning couple as the "natural" basis of parenthood.[48] Amrita Pande argues that Indian gestational surrogates claim kinship with the baby based on "shared blood" and gestational work.[49] They lay claims to motherhood while recognizing biological fathers' "property right" in the child.

While Israeli surrogates emphasize genetics and Indian surrogates highlight gestation to make sense of relatedness, in the United States both gestational and traditional surrogates see the fervent desire for a baby as the basis of parenthood. Kinship is reconceptualized as intent, desire, and love; yearning to be a parent is the "natural" basis of parenthood.[50] For US surrogates intent serves as a focal point for the emotional organization of motivation; they intend to make the intended parents' "dreams come true." Genetics, in surrogates' accounts, is simply material stuff, not what dreams are made of: "I guess I just don't see a difference in being an egg donor and being a TS, but I am very scientific and can view it as just DNA."

Surrogates' positions on these issues vary somewhat depending on the general thrust of the discussion. Some discussions highlight the difference between TS and GS, while others emphasize similarity. When women counter lay accusations of "baby selling" or lay questions such as "how can you give up your baby" or when they discuss their motivation, traditional and gestational surrogates agree that the baby was never theirs to begin with. The shared understanding is that biogenetics notwithstanding, "TS and GS do the same thing . . . we carry children for the intention of making a family that's not for ourselves."

However, in threads about TS versus GS decisions, gestational surrogates often say they could not do a traditional journey: "I would feel as if I am giving up a part of myself." Many others echoed this feeling. Gestational surrogates are careful never to imply that traditional surrogates "give up" their own children; they often make admiring comments about how traditional surrogates are "amazing" and give more of themselves. "What a wonderful gift, giving a piece of yourself!" "Giving someone a piece of yourself, in addition to your time and womb, is a very big deal!" "I look up to the TSs on this board and I highly respect them for doing such a selfless thing." Not being able to do traditional surrogacy is often presented as a personal limitation. "I know my limits. I think TS is one of the most wonderful things a person can do and kudos to those who can do it." "I guess what it comes down to is that some people (like you) have a bigger heart than most. Some people are givers."

There are other differences among traditional surrogates; those who carried for intended fathers sometimes express relatedness in ways that those who have heterosexual IPs never do:

> When we are together, I get to play mommy to him (though I leave all the changing for them!) and hand him back over to his daddies when I leave. We all went into that journey with me being known as the baby's mommy (since it was going to be obvious early on that there is a mommy somewhere). I know that many don't agree with this. . . . It was what all of us wanted, which was why we were a perfect match.

Even though Alyssa, above, explains her arrangement as a private decision made by the people involved in the relationship, "playing mommy" is not an option for traditional surrogates with heterosexual IPs. A surrogate who had carried for both gay and straight IPs reflected on the difference: "Where I don't mind my IFs children calling me mom, since they have no other mom, my IM is C.'s mom. . . .[My IM] dreamed of her forever and loved her before I met her." The following example shows how even though some traditional surrogates who had carried for intended fathers let their surrogate children call them "mommy," this is by no means common practice. In the following passage Candy, unlike Alyssa, spoke not only for herself but for traditional surrogates in general:

> I'm one of the TS that does acknowledge a TS babe is mine in the biological sense but he/she isn't MY baby. My babies are the ones I hug, kiss, cuddle, hold a bucket for when they are sick, who drive me absolutely mad with their attitudes sometimes, and who I make all decisions for together with DH. My TS babies have someone else who does all that stuff for them. Even now being matched with IFs I am still NOT THE MAMA!!! . . . We grow these babies, they are our biological link when it's TS but we are not their mothers. . . . No matter how long you babysit the child is never yours.

Kinship reorientation

A short post summarizes SMO agreement: "It doesn't matter if it is TS or GS, you are the surrogate." However, surrogates ponder relatedness beyond parenthood: "I don't think of my surrochildren as . . . my children's siblings." Kay explained her view with reference to the social relationship between family members: "Of course, there is that bio connection between a TS baby and your own child. I am not denying that fact. But when it comes down to it, my DS [darling son] is not referring to T (my surro son) as his brother. Why? Because T does not live with us, DS isn't doing sibling-like things for/with T, DS isn't seeing me mothering T."

Gestational surrogates who cannot imagine doing traditional surrogacy sometimes see it the opposite way: "I know I couldn't separate my emotions—that my kids would have a brother or sister out there. It's the biological connection that I couldn't get over. I have much respect for TSes but I know that I couldn't manage doing that." Some other gestational surrogates echoed this concern: "I'm a GS because I could not see myself being able to give up a part of my son, which I would see any baby—of my own, genetically—to be . . . his sibling, a piece of him. I couldn't do that. So . . . that's why I'm a GS."

These shifts from motherhood to siblinghood reveal the importance of a fuller relational context of third-party reproduction; it is two families rather than simply individuals that are involved. The surrogate's own children are the product of her own marriage, and their conception symbolizes the relationship between her and her husband.[51] Surrogates' reasoning indicates that the unity of this nuclear family would be threatened by having one's children's genetic siblings be part of another family. Peletz argued for "greater attention to the ways in which siblingship serves as a key symbol" and as a potential for relocating kinship in practice.[52]

Surrogates' posts testify to such a reorientation and relocation of kinship ties in third-party reproductive practices. Their accounts help us understand "social actors or the myriads of contexts in which they organize themselves, relate to one another, acquire and use resources, or create order and meaning in their lives."[53] Surrogates thus refashion as well as uphold the meaning of relatedness as a way to organize ties within their own families and with the families they help create and also, importantly, to distinguish between them. Intended mothers also engage in creative kinship reorientations:

> We plan on telling our little ones how much they were wanted, and the story of their conception (we drove for 24 hours straight so the doctor could mix the ingredients!) and how their Tummy Mommy

carried them and gave birth to them for us. Since we are doing TS, the genetics of the child will come into play sooner or later. . . . Our child will always know who their Tummy Mommy is. . . . We hope to remain in contact with our surrogate's family, so that the connection is strong while the child is growing up—I think of having a surrogate as being able to pick your own sister—probably cheesy, but how I feel.

SMO-ers love "going for sisters" with their intended mothers, and posts like the above are always warmly received. Clearly, the above IM's post does more than appreciate the surrogate; it relocates kinship from the relatedness between the traditional surrogate and the child to the fictive relatedness between the two women. Several surrogates I exchanged e-mails with described their IMs this way, too. "She is like a sister to me. . . . This is why I have offered them baby #3 recently," wrote Lori.[54] By framing the relationship as sisterhood, surrogates assume basic social equality with IPs.[55] SMO examples illuminate another interesting aspect of the relationship between surrogate and intended mother: at best, it establishes a chosen sisterhood, with the child as a link between the women. The biogenetic (GS) or biological-gestational (TS) link between the surrogate and the child is replaced by the fictive kinship the two women enact in their relationship. Thus, choice and action are equally important in creating both babies and relationships.

The only "negative case" I have encountered was Petra's distressed call for help; she "couldn't stop crying," she was missing her baby so much. "Was this an adoption? It sure doesn't sound like surrogacy," read the first response. "Did you go through the psych eval?" asked the next post. Petra did not offer too many details in her few responses, but SMO-ers puzzled out what happened. Based on the known facts, they pieced together the story: Petra was a first time TS who never was psychologically evaluated and, without "doing her homework," jumped into an independent arrangement with a gay couple. This explanation made Petra's emotional distress understandable to surrogates, and her case exemplified everything they disagree with. They concluded that this was not really adoption, but not really surrogacy, either.

No traditional surrogate, not even those who "play mommy" or say they are the mother of their surrogate children ever claimed that these surrogate children belong to them, and this unites surrogates on SMO. This is why Petra's post was received with such puzzlement, and even though women felt sorry for her, she was not considered a "real surrogate." Surrogate babies belong to their parents, whose love and desire for them, even if not their genetics, make them the only parents. Women who share this view are the real surrogates of the SMO community.

"I bonded with my IPs"

Bonding

Surrogates' attachment to their couple is informed by the same factors—planning the pregnancy, accepting responsibility, thinking of the fetus as an independent entity, and accommodating the pregnancy—that the literature found central to maternal bonding. "We bond more with the couples than the babies!! . . . Surrogacy is in no way just about growing a baby it is about . . . caring for the parents to be. . . . Our friendship doesn't end at birth." Surrogates conclude, "most people outside of surrogacy don't get [it]. Of course I'm interested in their child, but I'm more interested in them!"

Posts in the early 2000s often revealed that surrogates themselves were somewhat surprised at their own reaction: "Frankly after carrying triplets I was far more physically relieved than anything else. . . . I was very surprised by how sad I was to leave the parents at the hospital. In many ways I was more bonded with my IM." Over time, SMO-ers have come to take it for granted that "the bond I have isn't for the baby—but for its parents." Since they increasingly often anticipate bonding with the couple early on, they discuss the possible adverse consequences of attachment: "I'm afraid that if [the match falls apart] I have to start over and I will already be attached to them so I am trying to filter my emotions. How did you handle your feelings of wanting to jump in feet first but maintain a little distance to protect yourself?" Advice from others confirmed the emotional risk but also that it is worth taking:

> It is hard. I was recently matched, then it fell through a few days ago and I was so crushed because I really liked her a lot and thought she was the perfect match for me. . . . However, I don't regret letting down my guard at all, because that is the only way you can really get to know someone. You can't be too afraid of getting hurt emotionally, because you will never let yourself make these relationships otherwise.

Surrogates form emotional connection either with their couple as a unit or with the IM.[56] The following poignant post directly evokes mutual love: "Most people think you will have trouble giving up the baby . . . but the baby isn't mine from the beginning so that was nothing. But my intended parents were mine . . . and I was theirs also."[57] Many surrogates call their IM their "best friend." Intended fathers are the focus of bonding only when they are gay. For example, Cori was very openly emotional at the thought of parting with her gay couple. "I have become so attached to my IFs and will miss them terribly." Heterosexual intended fathers are never discussed this way, which is understandable, given the adulterous connotations of procreation outside of marriage.[58] Surrogates with heterosexual IPs tend to feel uncomfortable interacting with the intended father only and like it best when they "click" with the intended mother. "I feel very ready to let this little girl go home with her parents, and be a part of her real family. I am NOT ready to lose my IM. I feel bonded to her," wrote Nicolette.

The emotional connection surrogates feel or wish to feel to their couple is easier to understand if we consider that surrogacy involves the giving of oneself that in the modern Western cultural context is appropriate only in loving personal relationships.[59] Surrogates give themselves because being pregnant affects every aspect of one's daily life and involves potential risks. "Surrogacy is so intimate that it seems hard to envision a journey where you carry a child for IPs and you don't become friends or like family." Jenny could not imagine "not being friends" with her IPs, either: "Surrogacy is like dating. It is intimate and deeply personal and at times very invasive."[60] As one surrogate explained: "when people (strangers) ask me 'oh, are you doing it for a friend?' I always want to say yes. I mean, we are friends NOW."

Surrogates often want to do a "sibling project" for IPs they love. When the couple is undecided or unwilling, some surrogates are troubled by the thought of carrying for a new couple. "I almost felt weird trying to do it again, like dating so quickly after a spouse's death. I know it's not the right analogy but it's the one I can relate it to." All the responses were sympathetic, assuring this surrogate that what she felt was "completely natural." Several women responded in ways that were very similar to Ida's reaction: "I could not do it because I could not share *that* with anyone else." Many SMO-ers who felt this way eventually matched with new IPs, but women often deemed it important to get their former IPs' "blessing on the new journey."

The imagery of love and dating is widely used, yet only one traditional surrogate, Carly, confessed that after the birth she "started to feel attracted to and to have romantic feelings for" her former intended father:

I wondered before starting my surrogacy, how I would feel about another man whose child I carried and gave birth to. Now my question has been answered. I see now that surrogacy does carry with it, potential deep issues and problems considering the nature of what SMs and IPs are doing. What in life is more intimate and emotional than creating a child? I am left wondering how all the IFs (granted many are gay) come to feel about the woman who carries and gives birth to the child that they and their wives otherwise could never have had. Do they all feel nothing but platonic affection and gratitude?

Carly assured everyone that she was not trying to "stir up trouble" and did not expect support but felt obligated to write about her feelings. "I think it is only right that anyone considering surrogacy should be educated and aware of real potential issues, so they can make an informed decision."

Contrary to her expectation, her post was well received. Responses were mostly sympathetic, and some even expressed admiration for her courage to bring her story to the boards. Some speculated that Carly must have issues in her marriage if she fell in love with another man and urged her to attend to those problems. Others said they understood how attractive it was to see a man so deeply care about his wife that he would do surrogacy to make her a mother, and this feeling may be easy to confuse with love. The following harsh response was an exception: "You didn't go into surrogacy looking to fall in love and if you did something's wrong with you. You went into this to help create a family for another couple not to end a family."

However, other women ventured to say that this is probably not the only time such a thing happened; they also pointed out that people are not fully in control of their feelings, only whether they act on them or not. Carly's post revealed that she had carefully examined her feelings and framed the problem not simply as a personal one but as a potential issue for others and a topic worthy of discussion on SMO and was thus treated with respect and empathy.

Disappointments

Emotional attachment to IPs makes women vulnerable to disappointment. While there are couples and surrogates who develop a lasting friendship, many others have only sporadic contact. Women who are satisfied with their journey and the contact after birth typically post much less and less often, although they may briefly report new updates from their IPs. But posts about disappointments tend to be longer, and fellow surrogates frequently offer their stories for comfort; "bad stories" may thus be overrepresented. Surrogates repeatedly try to balance threads about bad outcomes with calls for competing threads of good stories. However, threads labeled "great surrogacy journeys" tend to peter out quickly. Good journeys do not make good stories; "a story begins with a breach in the expected state of things. . . . Something goes awry, otherwise there is nothing to tell about."[61]

In some cases, the relationship sours even before the journey is over. There are IPs who do not initiate communication and do not go to appointments during the pregnancy, do not return calls and e-mails or respond only briefly. Women frequently give IPs the benefit of the doubt, saying that after so much heartbreak, IPs must be cautious and "guard their hearts against further disappointments." They advise one another to "give IPs time" and respect their need for emotional distance; they express hope that as the pregnancy proceeds, the couple will relax. Another IP-friendly argument centers on the unpredictability of personal relationships during major life changes: "Giving most IPs the benefit of the doubt, they may not know how their feelings or focus may change. None of us know what's around the corner after a life changing event."[62]

Annie, like so many others in similar situations, looked for support after she "tried everything" to make her relationship with her IPs better. "Emails are rarely answered and if they are they are one liners. Why keep trying? Why keep giving so much of myself emotionally to get nothing in return? I am not one who wants a daily phone call or even gifts of thanks. Her happiness would be enough thanks." Fellow surrogates rallied: "Know that YOU are doing an amazing thing NO MATTER how you are being treated and have been misled. I don't think IMs realize how much we NEED to feel their happiness and joy to get through these pregnancies. Maybe some do but I know a LOT just can't seem to grasp it." Responses acknowledged the hurt but refocused attention to the goal: the babies and the families. "It's so sad that we put so much of ourselves into a pregnancy that even the parents don't seem to appreciate . . . but, as you have pointed out, the health and wellbeing of the babies, and of course bringing them into this world to be with their parents (although seemingly ungrateful), is what is most important."

In the following response to Annie, a fellow surrogate shifts the focus from her own disappointment to the IPs' insecurity and "fear" of surrogates' power to create life:

> I too feel i am a good judge of people, but how can you judge people or get to know the real person through lies?? You can't. They simply tell you what you want to hear. They know you are a good person . . . if not would they really have chosen you to carry their children? No. All they want is their baby. . . . It was hard the first few months after birth. I felt as if i was dying. But i finally just came to realize that, i think they are so scared of us . . . of doing what they can't.

The SMO consensus is that "so many odd behaviors rest on insecurities and infertility." Such shifts recontextualize the problem as one of insecurity, and even though the IPs' behavior still pains the surrogate, she is able to cherish the power of her fertility and generosity. These narrative shifts illuminate surrogates' discursive use of the abilities they take pride in such as their fertility and willingness to sacrifice.

Pointing to IPs' failings or ingratitude does not mean that SMO-ers condone retaliation in any way. A revealing example of this sentiment is from the thread Joanna started. Her relationship had "severely deteriorated" over disagreement about financial issues.

> For those of you whose relationship went way sour during the pregnancy, how did you cope? . . . It's affecting me tremendously 😔. . .
>
> Of course, most of it surrounds financial concerns. Disputes over what they are obligated to pay. . . . I've tried to be very fair and not ask for anything other than what is detailed in the contract. I've even conveyed that I don't even care about the money anymore. If they want to argue over a few hundred dollars and destroy our relationship over it, that's sad. . . . Deep inside, I'm disappointed that they are disputing their clear obligations so cold heartedly, and even though I don't care about the money anymore, the damage has been done because it shows what kind of people they are, and how they view this arrangement—as a business arrangement. . . . They have emotionally distanced themselves from the relationship. And it's in stark contrast to how things were in the beginning. . . . they talked of how they would always think of us as extended family. . . . a business arrangement is NOT what I have ever wanted.

Sympathetic responses advised Joanna to focus on the twins she was carrying and urged her to take care of herself. Personal stories similar to hers were offered for consolation and advice:

I focused on the pregnancy and my "task at hand" since I'm a goal oriented person. My job regardless of what FIM was doing, was to gestate a healthy, calm and peaceful pregnancy to give her daughter the best possible start to life. And so I took care of myself, focused on the fact that the innocent little girl I was carrying didn't have any say and so I had to be her advocate. . . . I learned how great of things we can accomplish regardless of the amount of stress, pain and chaos another individual can put you through. She will turn 4 next month and I've never heard a peep from them, but I am fully healed and content with how everything happened. I set out to help a woman become a mother, I didn't set out to make best friends, have my hand held or be coddled. . . . I birthed a beautiful, precious little child and made one woman's dream come true of becoming a mother. That's all that matters and all I had set out to do.

The solution advocated—one that is given increasingly often in cases like Joanna's—is to concentrate on the ultimate goal of surrogacy: a healthy pregnancy and creating a family. SMO-ers maintain that poor treatment from IPs is always a test of character. Those who unwaveringly keep their promise to nurture the baby and stay focused on this goal accomplish a "great thing" and pass the test with flying colors. Embarking on a new journey can also be healing, as women who had been through similar disappointments point out: "I'm over it now—it's only time that heals, and surprisingly a new journey and new IPs."

Wendy was upset not only because her relationship with her couple deteriorated but also because they denied her request to hold and say goodbye to the twins after birth. Fellow surrogates urged her to explain to her IPs that this would give her the closure she needed. Miriam's advice was an exception; it contradicted the SMO consensus that surrogates should never respond in kind to IPs' unreasonable or bad behavior:

I would . . . assert my control . . . and hold the babies if that was my desire. After all you did carry them. . . . It's not like being nice and doing everything they want will save the relationship. I know people get flamed all the time for saying this but here goes . . . I wouldn't invite them to the birth.

SMO-ers were outraged at Miriam's suggestion: "a baby isn't a thing to use against someone else to even a painful score." Responses passionately took issue with her advice:

I can't sit by silently and read another surrogate advocating to hold
the baby hostage for a few hours after birth. . . . Sure you'll get to
hold and say goodbye to the baby, but if you have a heart and feelings the guilt will eat you up because you aren't just taking that
time away from IPs (which is rightfully theirs as the parent and not
yours as a surrogate) but you're also taking those precious moments
away from the child to bond and be in their parents' arms . . . with
how rocky and awful the end of my journey was . . . [still] I wanted
her . . . to . . . take on the role as mother. . . . No matter what a person
does to me or [how she] treats me, child and mother deserve to have
those unforgettable first moments with each other.

Other responses to Miriam's advice also upheld the same surrogacy
ethic:

if we aren't able to accept that things don't always end the way we
want and what's most important is the babies' well-being (including
emotional) maybe we have no business being surrogates. . . . I've seen
and lived the worst case scenario and can hold my head high knowing that I respected the child that was put in the middle of a horrific
situation, and I can tell you the healing that comes from that surpasses
the petty desire to give a tit for tat or to have my way or the highway.

Responses reflect the notion that surrogates' moral superiority is
rooted not simply in altruistic giving but in the unwavering dedication to the goal: to provide the best environment for the "IPs'
baby" and facilitate the bonding between the parents and their
child, no matter how the journey ends. "Yes they are growing in
you. But they are not yours. Not in any way." The general consensus is that IPs have all the parental rights even if they mistreat
their surrogate and refuse to pay what was agreed in the contract.
Anyone who suggests retaliation should be prepared to be a social
pariah on SMO. Women underline their dedication and perform
their moral superiority vis-à-vis both dishonest IPs and revengeful
surrogates.

Danielle pointed out that "it's important to remember . . . that like
a marriage, we never go into this expecting the relationship to go
downhill." But as many anguished stories indicate, some relationships do go downhill even before the birth, and contact with IPs
tends to decrease afterward. Surrogates often report a sense of loss
and sadness: "I can feel our relationship changing. The calls are less
often and shorter. The distance has begun." SMO discussions build
acceptance and resignation: "There is nothing wrong with feeling
pain during or after surrogacy. LOVE is painful, no?" Jess tried to

prepare a fellow surrogate to the phase after birth: "I bonded more with my IPs . . . I miss my IPs . . . the baby . . . is NOT the loss that I grieved. Your relationship most certainly does change." Women often give the couple the benefit of the doubt, saying that IPs are busy with their new baby, "their hands are full," but it is hard to ignore the question many women raise: "it took more than a year of my life to give them a baby; how long does it take to shoot me a short e-mail?"

Deceptions and hurt feelings

Continued contact is not primarily a question of time, as some IPs make clear: "we want to continue to work towards some level of closure with you." Others are less civil and ask the surrogate not to contact them ever again, and some others "drop off from the face of the earth." There are IPs who change their telephone number and e-mail address or set the surrogate's as spam; some "unfriend" their surrogate on Facebook. Surrogates often conclude that "some couples lie and tell the surro what she wants to hear during the journey."[63] SMO-ers often discuss the role of expectations: "a lot of us go into this with rose-colored glasses—especially with our first times, myself included. It ended very differently than I originally hoped."

Even though "business deal" and "employee" always have negative connotation in SMO posts, surrogates do not condemn IPs who explicitly want a "business deal." Surrogates who post on the subject say that they personally would not want such an arrangement and that it may take longer for these IPs to match. The only surrogates who say they would consider "a business deal" for future journeys had IPs who went back on their promises. Yet reading such threads has not convinced me that these women would truly welcome a "business arrangement."

Their alleged willingness to enter into one seems more like a strategy to avoid leaving themselves vulnerable to betrayal: "At least I would know up front what the IPs wanted or did not want, as opposed to lie to me as my IPs did," explained Margie. "I hate to say it, but if I attempt another surrogacy, it will be very business-like. I would rather have a few people think poorly of me then to have my feelings hurt again and again," wrote Lynn.

SMO-ers, who in the early 2000s condemned "the business of surrogacy," no longer do so, although most say they would not enter such an arrangement. What they do condemn is deception and dishonesty. "It would be nice if IPs were honest about what they

wanted out of a relationship instead of stringing their SM along, but
we all know this isn't the case for many people."

> I think that it would be very hard to find a surrogate who didn't want
> contact afterward. To go through a year or longer of . . . medications,
> pregnancy and then the birth and then to never hear from the IPs
> again? It happens all the time, unfortunately. But it's not planned
> that way. IPs tell the surrogates that they will keep in touch. . . .
> Sometimes a journey will go bad. . . . Other times the IPs just had no
> intention of updating, they just said they did. It is extremely hurtful
> to be the surrogate in a situation like that. They feel like they were
> used and tossed aside.[64]

It is this potential for deception and betrayal that makes surrogates uneasy. "This time, I've tried to guard my heart a little
more, and watch that I not become too attached to my IPs," posted
Joan, whose first journey unexpectedly ended badly. Sympathetic
responses emphasized how hard it is to trust again after one's heart
was broken. Dissenting advice, on the other hand, encouraged her
to put the past behind her. "I tend to wear my heart on my sleeve
and deal with the hurt when it comes . . . but it's my opinion that if
you guard yourself from your current IPs just because of what your
FIPs did . . . you may be missing out on something wonderful." On
SMO realism does not preclude optimism: "if you have to deal with
them being fair-weather at the end then deal with it then. They
are going to be the way they are no matter how you are. . . . So I
say be happy, throw yourself into if you want to and enjoy these
moments!!!"
Generally, however, surrogates want IPs to be truthful and not
make promises they do not intend to keep: "All a surrogate wants
is what is promised to her in the beginning." Women want their
couple to tell them "their 'REAL' plans for our future relationship or
lack of. . . . I need a couple that is genuine when they say that they
want to be friends forever." But as this and many other posts indicate, surrogates want more than simple honesty and may not want
to carry for couples who honestly do not want any contact after
birth. SMO-ers wish that IPs had an honest desire to be "friends
forever." This desire is consistent with the framing of surrogacy as
a "labor of love" and "the gift of life," as I will discuss in Chapter 5.
Surrogates often struggle to "hold their head high" in some other
difficult and often shockingly surprising situations as well. Some
IPs work with more than one surrogate without telling either, and
the accidental discovery comes as a shock: "Has anyone else come

across this? . . . I feel very betrayed right now. The other surro and I have been talking for a little while, and when she was telling me more, I come to find out that she was talking to my IPs." Fellow surrogates reassured her that this was not right even if the IM "was just hedging her bets," and they, too, would "feel awful." Several women explained that it was the lying that was wrong: "I would feel super betrayed! If they wanted to look for another surro, they should have been open and honest with you as soon as they made their decision." Even those who had no personal experience were insistent on one point: "The whole key to surrogacy is trusting one another." The advice about how to "confront the IPs" also underlined the importance of trust: "you need to have complete trust without any secrets with your Intended Parents." Sometimes women do not find out about the other surrogate until after the birth:

> Would it hurt your feelings if you found out AFTER DELIVERY, your IPs had a 2nd surrogate who gave birth a week before you did? and THEN when you asked them POINT BLANK about it, the IM lied to your face? . . . I had started shaking. . . . it hurt my feelings that she hid it from me. . . . I started crying because I felt deceived. . . . I just felt like after EVERYTHING I've been through [with twins], and how awful the last month has been here. . . . I almost died this last delivery and put MY LIFE at risk for them, they lied to me about it.

Another woman found two babies instead of one at the IPs' house when she dropped off breast milk for her surrogate baby: "First I was confused, but then I felt very hurt, even betrayed." Most of the women who responded said they would not want to carry for such IPs, but for the vast majority, dishonesty was the deal breaker. "I feel these journeys are like our marriages. It's all about trust and honesty. And when you find out someone was not you feel betrayed." However, surrogates were sympathetic to IPs' quest for maximizing the chances of pregnancy and understood why some of them may be in a hurry to complete their family. A few women even said this just confirmed how much they wanted to be parents, which, to SMO-ers, confirms that they are deserving IPs. Yet no one said that these considerations excused dishonesty and deception. "There are plenty of surros that have no issue with dual surrogacy. Why not be upfront and honest. . . . I've heard of this [lying about a second surrogate] happening many times and it always amazes me."

However, even though SMO-ers are generally sympathetic to IPs who openly want to work with two surrogates, quite a few women listed possible problems that would deter them from entering into such an arrangement. "What if the other GS gets pregnant first?" was one of the frequently raised questions. "I am committed to my IPs ~ meaning I will try as long as they want. It is A LOT for a GS to go through, all the appts, all the meds, etc. . . . for the IPs to drop you if the other GS is prego and you are not. I've invested lots of time getting to know my IPs." Although surrogates support IPs' quest for children, they sometimes worry that their investment in the relationship and efforts to make them parents could easily be devalued if the couple has more than one surrogate. Women address the potential emotional roller coaster that a nonexclusive relationship may entail even as they agree that the goal is to create a baby and a family rather than a good relationship.

Discussing these potential complications has its own complications; surrogates are cautious not to come across as needy of attention and appreciation. As a result, they focus on their emotional as well as time commitment to IPs rather than their fear that IPs would be less grateful and appreciative if they had two surrogates. When an IM whose "clock was ticking" posted about her plan to find two surrogates with the intention of being honest about it and following through with both, she found support on the boards. Surrogates told her that her case was "completely different"; the surrogates' time and effort would not be wasted since she promised to "keep going" until both were pregnant. Tactfully, the question of appreciation was not raised.

Losses

Discussions reveal that failed conceptions and pregnancy loss are experienced as painful and traumatic events. Surrogates grieve, remember, and commemorate losses; yet, as I have documented before, they disclaim attachment to the fetus. Exploring loss narratives reveals interconnected feelings of failure and responsibility, the effort invested in creating and nurturing life, and the desire to give the gift of life and make couples' "dreams come true." Clifford Geertz argued that a "good interpretation of anything . . . takes us into the heart of that of which it is an interpretation."[65] Surrogates' grieving accounts of loss, on closer scrutiny, take us into the heart of surrogacy: the relationship between surrogates and intended parents and surrogates' promise to make IPs parents.

Although surrogates acknowledge that every pregnancy is different and involves risks beyond their control, their sense of agency is often quite striking.[66] "I have learned that I know my body much better than the doctors. I felt that I could be pregnant successfully again and I was. I wanted to be able to give the gift of parenthood to another couple and I did that." Even when surrogates talk about fertility and pregnancy as a "blessing," that is, as a fortunate event for which they cannot take full credit, they are determined to "share" it with their couple and "make people's dreams come true." My contention is that when surrogates lay claim to agency in achieving pregnancy, they leave themselves more vulnerable to failure and loss. This, however, seems inevitable; they put much thought and physical and emotional effort into the enterprise of carrying someone else's baby and persevere after failed attempts, and in this sense their active role is undeniable. Reproductive technologies contribute to a sense of loss by holding out the hope of successful outcome if people are willing to "do what it takes" to have a baby. Scholars of assisted reproductive technologies have described how these technologies create new hopes, dilemmas, and desires.[67]

What I will, for the sake of simplicity, call "loss" is in fact a range of events or nonevents from failed conceptions and embryo transfer cycles through chemical pregnancy[68] to miscarriage, premature labor, and stillbirth. The following posts illustrate this range. "We had 3 losses with my previous IPs: a miscarriage at 6 weeks, 6 days, a chemical pregnancy at 5 weeks, 2 days, and our last miscarriage at 14 weeks, 2 days." Another surrogate, trying to conceive for an older couple, reported that "after 2 canceled cycles because our IM could no longer produce any eggs to retrieve we parted ways as IPs/SM. I was so upset for their loss." By most accounts canceled or failed cycles are considered to be "losses."

Sometimes such losses are compared to death. An intended mother posted the following response to a surrogate whose failed transfer upset her IPs, "I can tell you that a failed cycle can feel as bad as a death in a family. (I've had people tell me, 'You can't mean that . . .') But it's a really personal thing. And it did hurt that bad." Surrogates frequently agree: "When you're trying to conceive and it doesn't work, it feels like a miscarriage. . . . The assumption is that you're pregnant, so when you find out you're not expecting a baby, it feels like somebody has died."

At times, surrogates are more devastated than their intended parents: "With my last IPs I had a failed cycle and cried and cried and my IPs didn't. She explained it to me that they have had so much disappointment that they are always prepared for the worst, and pray for the best. So they were prepared for a failed cycle or a loss. I wasn't." Marie was equally unprepared: "I never imagined the pain & let down that I feel now! and to think that is nothing compared

to the pain my IPs are probably feeling!!!" Surrogates readily agree
that failed conceptions "are heart breakers :(BIG ((HUGS)) to you
and your IPs!" Losses "in the heart" then parallel "conceptions in
the heart."[69] Conceptions that fail to develop into viable pregnancies are also most often described as "heartbreaking," as are miscarriages. Josie summed up the majority view: "YES, you mourn
the loss of a child at any stage of gestation!"

There are some striking similarities in the narrative accounts
of these different events called loss by surrogates. "Baby," "child,"
"death," and "heartbreak" are some of the most frequently used
words in threads about loss. In order to make sense of surrogates'
emotional response and understand how these disparate events
call forth similar reactions, we need to remember that surrogates
most frequently consider not only fetuses but also fertilized ova as
"baby in different stages of development." Not infrequently, though,
IPs' desire for a baby is considered the real beginning of personhood, and surrogates see themselves as babysitters with heightened
responsibility for the babies entrusted to their care.

These ideas create specific hurdles for surrogates. Failure to produce the baby is often emotionally crushing for them. They are also
sympathetic to the loss they think the couple feels and often match
the intensity of the couple's perceived sorrow. Some intended mothers express extreme grief, while others do not communicate their
feelings; yet surrogates almost always assume that the couple is
devastated. "I can only image how they feel." Imagination plays a
large and important role in surrogates' understanding of loss and
informs their responses to it.

The contention that intended parents suffer more is supported
by intended parents, mostly mothers, whose posts resonate deeply
with surrogates. "I am very sorry about the miscarriage and what
you went through, I'm sure you hurt and I know you wanted the
best for your IPs but they JUST suffered a HUGE, HUGE loss (it
happened to me once with a GS at 8 weeks). They are probably not
ready to deal, communicate, thank you or stop grieving right now,"
wrote an intended mother. When Ariel complained that after the
failed transfer she barely had contact with her intended mother, an
IM explained that "another neg[ative] is devastating . . . WHY ME.
Each neg means another piece of our dream is gone, another piece
of our heart / our hopes is gone."

It is a common argument that "losses in the heart" are forever
and are harder to bear than losses in the body. One intended mother,
who already had two children, reminded surrogates:

I am sorry that . . . you must experience pain and discomfort but please remember this isn't ALL about you. . . . You are having a miscarriage, yes, I realize that and it's miserable. . . . But please try to remember that is my baby that died inside your body. . . . life will be back to normal for you. . . . I will spend the rest of my life missing my unborn child. . . . My arms will ache for the rest of my life to hold that baby.

Surrogates are caught between two disturbing alternatives. If they identify with their couple's perceived suffering and feel responsible for "letting them down," they can lose themselves in grief. In rare instances, they remind the grief-stricken fellow surrogate: "Keep your chin up and take time to heal yourself. As surrogates I think we get wrapped up in the IPs' perspectives and tend to overlook the fact that we have just experienced a MISCARRIAGE." However, when they do not identify fully with their couple's perceived sense of loss, they may be called unsympathetic and self-centered by intended mothers and even fellow surrogates.

Surrogates' own accounts articulate the meaning of loss: it is the failure to give a baby to IPs who put their faith in them. "It was the most horrible, most painful experience ever. I'm . . . young and healthy and I couldn't give my IPs their miracle." Mourning the loss means grieving for the surrogacy dream of "making parents" and an attempt at sharing the IPs' anguish and affirming the shared nature of the journey. Losses often fuel surrogates' resolve to keep trying until they succeed.

"honor the journey"

Emotional regime

When I started to read SMO threads, surrogates whose "heart got broken" were typically comforted with wishes for a better match or better journeys in the future. Women still hope for this, but voices asserting that creating life is its own reward even if the IPs are unappreciative have been growing stronger. Surrogates remind one another to think of the "precious life that would not be here without you . . . no one will ever take that away from you."

This approach is the result of two developments: the collective lesson learned from numerous stories of disappointment and the crystallization of the shared definition of the purpose of surrogacy: "surrogacy is not about gaining new friends but about creating a family." Ava admitted that she had no idea what she would

have done had her IPs treated her the way many IPs treat their
surrogates.

> I think what you find behind the scenes is a lot of these surrogates
> take the time to focus on the life they've created instead of the loss
> they feel over the relationship with their IPs. . . . There comes a lot
> of strength from knowing that you have brought life into this world,
> even if it doesn't have that beautiful, picture perfect ending.[70]

There has been a distinctive shift toward a collective and vocal
affirmation that "it was all worth it." Paula offered the mantra she
learned from an experienced surrogate: "[She] reminded me that
there was a beautiful little girl in the world . . . and that in spite of
the pain I was feeling over the way it ended (for me), that I should
remember to honor the journey. That became my mantra. . . . I have
it tattooed in kanji on my ankle." A lot of surrogates struggle to fully
adopt this outlook.

> I learned the hard way that the idea of something is far more rosy
> and lovely than the reality. I gave a piece of my soul up to carry
> these babies and I feel I was taken advantage of. It has taken me two
> years to even get to the point of being able to talk about it. The thing
> I try to remember is that there are two little people in this world.
> Because I opened my heart to them. I just wish my heart hadn't been
> crushed in the process.

Yet the most sure way to overcome heartache and receive sympathy and praise is to embrace this new "emotional regime" by "letting
go of the negative feelings and seeing the positives—you helped
bring a child into the world."[71] The following sympathetic reply was
meant to console Connie, who felt "ditched" by her couple but was
nevertheless thinking of doing another surrogacy: "Surrogacy is
hard, trying . . . loving. . . . Surrogacy can make or break a person."
Such responses empathize with as well as express approval of the
surrogate who "had it in her heart" to look for IPs again and thus
was not broken by surrogacy.[72]

Marcy was one such disappointed, yet "unbroken" surrogate:
"I know that I have done the right thing and hopefully can help
another family out someday." She was praised for her accomplishment and resolve. "I'm sorry you're hurting. You did something so
wonderful and all you're left with is pain. Know that we're all here
loving you and supporting you. I think the most amazing thing is
that you're willing to put yourself out there again. That speaks vol-
umes as to the kind of person you are." A few IMs joined in support,

and their appreciation—and their implied criticism of IPs who do not value their surrogate—is highly prized on the boards: "you're not the first GS i've heard from who had this experience, but i just can't wrap my mind around it. i can't possibly imagine doing that to our GS . . . my heart hurts for you."

Moral meanings

By affirming that "it was all worth it," women are articulating a position that even unreciprocated love can lead to repeated giving: "in no way will I allow their selfishness and broken promises to deter me from another journey." This joint effort to "see the positives" allows women to uncouple surrogacy from specific journeys and uphold the value of surrogacy even in the face of bad experience. This approach insists that the love and empathy women feel for IPs is noble and ennobling and only "special women" are capable of this kind of giving. "In the end I know I am the BETTER person" is a sentiment expressed by many women on SMO who felt betrayed. Surrogates resort to "personal control" as a response to relationship troubles with IPs.[73] This, in turn, makes it possible to hold on to a sense of uniqueness even when IPs deny the personal and unique nature of the relationship.

In a rare post a very angry and bitter surrogate confessed regretting "ever meeting this couple." Others were clearly uncomfortable with this attitude and, rather than sympathizing with her, reminded her to focus on the "precious life" she had created. The consensus on SMO is that no matter what IPs say or do, surrogacy is a "labor of love," and one should not only never regret giving life but strive to continue to do so even in the face of ingratitude. With this emotional adjustment, lack of reciprocity achieves the same end as reciprocity: both bestow value on surrogates, albeit of a different kind. However, in the very few cases in which women publicly refused to make this adjustment and demanded contact, raising the possibility of a lawsuit as Olivia did, the SMO community was quick to condemn. "You're trying to blackmail them into an update or contact. . . . Personally, if I were them, I'd be freaked out and doing all I could to keep you out, too."

Women, especially experienced surrogates, present themselves as resourceful, knowledgeable, loving, and giving yet emotionally independent, wise, and outspoken with a good sense of humor; they have their "big girl panties on." This term has surfaced fairly recently and now women reference it in posts, and some include it in their siggy: "Cathy, working on pregnancy #3 if my uterus doesn't fall out. Excuse me if I show my bum. I pulled up my big-girl panties so much the elastic broke." Given the responses to "whiny" posts about IPs' betrayal, it is clearly advantageous to put on "big girl panties" if one hopes to receive praise and encouragement. SMO-ers consistently applaud women who suffer the pain of betrayal yet are able to move on: "there are no guarantees in life, surrogacy or otherwise. You need to make the best of whatever situation you are in."

Ella, who established herself as the voice of reason, told a disappointed surrogate that she, too, was "shut out" after the birth, but then through her attorney she advised her IPs to never contact her again. Thus, rather than feeling like a victim, she felt "liberated and free" and advised others to do the same. "I look at it this way—I opened the door in the beginning, I closed it in the end."

It is impossible to miss the performative flourish in the following post about not needing updates from IPs: "Am I the only one [who says] I have a life and it does not revolve around someone else's kid(s)?" On SMO, women discursively, interactively, and at times competitively perform, negotiate, and delineate emotional realities.[74] As Goffman observed, such performances "incorporate and exemplify officially accredited values" such as helpfulness, generosity, competence, and autonomy.[75] These performances also reveal surrogates' ideal, "truer" self: the self they collectively fashion and are collectively committed to.[76]

Sally, one of the experienced surrogate moderators, who carried eight surrogate babies, expressed this ideal self in her consoling response to Lisbeth, whose IPs not only had a second surrogate but blamed her for the deterioration of their relationship when she insisted on receiving the payment that was due to her:

> I know exactly what you mean Lisbeth. It hurts when we don't get the outcome that we would so desire as surrogates. That's why I can't stress enough that the match is THE MOST important thing in surrogacy. . . . Don't stop giving the love that you so want to give because it will come back to you in one form or another. Even the most perfect journey is never PERFECT! IPs obviously go into surrogacy with [the] intent of starting a family. Some will keep us in their lives and some will not. . . . I always trust my intuition. The beauty of assisting others in creating [a] family is beyond words for me. Many people just don't get . . . why we do what we do. . . . Some IMs just don't get over their infertility issues . . .
>
> I've been way down and out with surrogacy and have questioned myself a zillion times and it's always ONLY made me stronger.

Stronger as a woman, stronger as a mother and stronger as a friend. Don't give up just because of a few bad apples. If surrogacy is something of your passion, follow your heart but take your head along.

Tasha had her own letdowns but vowed to not give up on surrogacy: "I will not let my former IPs ruin surrogacy for me!" Distinguishing specific journeys from surrogacy as an ideal enables surrogates to uphold the beauty and value of the practice and also acknowledge hurt and disappointment at the same time.

According to SMO consensus, the ideal surrogate is giving and forgiving, intuitive and intelligent, sympathetic and independent. In her quest to better other people's lives, she also becomes a better person who emerges from disappointments with renewed resolve. Underlying these ideals is the understanding that while reproduction is a biological process and thus morally neutral, reproductive actions are the outcome of choices that carry moral meanings. Surrogates maintain that surrogacy is possible not simply because of advances in reproductive technologies but because a self-selected group of caring women chooses to gestate and birth babies for others.

Notes

1. Heléna Ragoné, *Surrogate Motherhood: Conceptions in the Heart* (Boulder, CO: Westview, 1994), 67.
2. Ibid., 58.
3. In a poll that asked, "Would you do a journey if your mom (dad, etc.) was against it?" Ninety percent of the close to one hundred women who responded said yes and only five percent said no.
4. Kara, e-mail communication, 3 June 2003.
5. Joy, e-mail communication, 15 May 2003.
6. Elly Teman, *Birthing a Mother: The Surrogate Body and the Pregnant Self* (Berkeley: University of California Press, 2010), 68.
7. See Robert Bellah et al., *Habits of the Heart: Individualism and Commitment in American Life* (Berkeley: University of California Press, 1985), 89; Eva Illouz, *Consuming the Romantic Utopia: Love and the Cultural Contradictions of Capitalism* (Berkeley: University of California Press, 1997); David M. Schneider, *American Kinship: A Cultural Account* (Englewood Cliffs, NJ: Prentice-Hall, 1968).
8. Aaron Ben-Ze'ev, *The Subtlety of Emotions* (Cambridge, MA: MIT Press, 2000); Robert Solomon, *About Love: Reinventing Romance for Our Times* (New York: Simon and Schuster, 1988).
9. Schneider, *American Kinship*.

10. George Lakoff and Mark Johnson, *Metaphors We Live By* (Chicago: University of Chicago Press, 2008), 97–105.
11. Arthur W. Frank, *The Wounded Storyteller: Body, Illness, and Ethics* (Chicago: University of Chicago Press, 1995), 117. Frank contends that Campbell's book "profoundly affected the narrative presuppositions" of journey narratives.
12. Ragoné, *Surrogate Motherhood,* 41–43.
13. Elizabeth F.S. Roberts, "Examining Surrogacy Discourses between Feminine Power and Exploitation," in *Small Wars: The Cultural Politics of Childhood,* ed. N. Scheper-Hughes and C. Sargent (Berkeley: University of California Press, 1998), 197.
14. Ava, e-mail communication, 26 April 2010.
15. Karen Lystra, *Searching the Heart: Women, Men, and Romantic Love in Nineteenth-Century America* (New York: Oxford University Press, 1989), 32–35.
16. Kathy, e-mail communication, 4 March 2010.
17. Teman, *Birthing a Mother,* 264.
18. Lisa, e-mail communication, 6 April 2003.
19. Robert Solomon, *About Love: Reinventing Romance for Our Times* (New York: Simon & Schuster, 1988); Lystra, *Searching the Heart.*
20. Jodi, e-mail communication, 19 October 2004.
21. Solomon makes a similar point about love in *About Love,* 36–37.
22. Lakoff and Johnson, *Metaphors We Live By,* 150, 154.
23. Sophie, e-mail communication, 2 June 2010.
24. William H. Sewell, Jr., "The Concept(s) of Culture," in *Beyond the Cultural Turn: New Directions in the Study of Society and Culture,* ed. V.E. Bonnell and L. Hunt (Berkeley: University of California Press, 1999), 51.
25. Tessa, online surrogacy diary. Tessa included the link to her online diary under her siggy, and fellow surrogates followed her journey and its aftermath. When, following her surrogacy, Tessa got pregnant and then went into early labor with her third child, who died shortly after the birth, SMO-ers collected money for a present for Tessa.
26. Linda L. Layne, "'He was a Real Baby with Baby Things' A Material Culture Analysis of Personhood, Parenthood and Pregnancy Loss." *Journal of Material Culture* 5, no. 3 (2000): 322.
27. Nicole N. Isaacson, "The 'Fetus-Infant': Changing Classifications of in Utero Development in Medical Texts," *Sociological Forum* 11, no. 3 (1996): 457–80.
28. M.J. Casper, "Reframing and Grounding Nonhuman Agency: What Makes a Fetus an Agent?" *American Behavioral Scientist* 37, no. 6 (1994): 839–56.
29. http://www.fetalcarecenter.org/fetal-surgery/surgical-procedures/.
30. E.g., Susan E. Chase and Mary F. Rogers, *Mothers and Children: Feminist Analyses and Personal Narratives* (New Brunswick, NJ: Rutgers University Press, 2001); Martha A. Field, *Surrogate Motherhood* (Cambridge, MA: Harvard University Press, 1988); Christine Overall, *Ethics and*

Human Reproduction: A Feminist Analysis (Boston: Allen and Unwin, 1987).

31. Barbara K. Rothman, *Recreating Motherhood* (New York: WW Norton, 1989), 171.
32. Barbara K. Rothman, "Women as Fathers: Motherhood and Child Care under a Modified Patriarchy," *Gender & Society* 3, no. 1 (1989): 90.
33. Paul Lauritzen, *Pursuing Parenthood: Ethical Issues in Assisted Reproduction* (Bloomington: Indiana University Press, 1993), 109–10.
34. Jane Collier and Sylvia Yanagisako, "Toward a Unified Analysis of Gender and Kinship," in *Gender and Kinship: Essays toward a Unified Analysis* (Stanford: Stanford University Press, 1987), 32.
35. Gasking, qtd. in Melvin Pollner, "Mundane Reasoning," *Philosophy of the Social Sciences* 4, no. 1 (1974): 43.
36. Ibid., 44.
37. Nancy Scheper-Hughes, *Death without Weeping: The Violence of Everyday Life in Brazil* (Berkeley: University of California Press, 1993).
38. Marshall H. Klaus and John H. Kennell, *Maternal-Infant Bonding: The Impact of Early Separation or Loss on Family Development* (St-Louis: Mosby, 1976), 39.
39. Jane Collier, Michelle Z. Rosaldo, and Sylvia Yanagisako, "Is There a Family? New Anthropological Views," in *Rethinking the Family,* ed. Barrie Thorne with Marilyn Yalom (New York: Longman, 1982).
40. For a more comprehensive discussion, see Zsuzsa Berend, "'We Are All Carrying Someone Else's Child!': Relatedness and Relationships in Third-Party Reproduction," *American Anthropologist* 118 (2016):24-36.
41. Rene Almeling, *Sex Cells: The Medical Market for Eggs and Sperm* (Berkeley: University of California Press, 2010), 149–53.
42. Traditional surrogates often articulate their role the same way: "My surrobabe was intended for HIS parents from day one. I know that biologically he is mine, but I also view myself as the egg donor and the surrogate that carried him. I don't call him my surroson, because he's not my son. . . . I call him my surrobabe."
43. Lauritzen (*Pursuing Parenthood*) documented how fertility specialists present the various options in similar ways, as the road leading to the baby. The following description of the solutions fertility clinics offer is quite typical: "It is important to understand the philosophy with which the Jones Institute approaches the management and treatment of infertility. Here, our goal is to help couples achieve their dreams of having children" (http://www.jonesinstitute.org/ivf-success-rates.html). "Egg donation . . . can be used as an effective treatment for infertility," states the website of the Advanced Fertility Center of Chicago (http://www.advancedfertility.com/eggdonor.htm).
44. Sarah Franklin, "Making Miracles: Scientific Progress and the Facts of Life," in *Reproducing Reproduction: Kinship, Power, and Technological Innovation,* ed. Sarah Franklin and Heléna Ragoné (Philadelphia: University of Pennsylvania Press, 1998), 102.

45. Schneider, *American Kinship*, 1–27.
46. Marilyn Strathern, *Reproducing the Future: Essays on Anthropology, Kinship, and the New Reproductive Technologies* (New York: Routledge, 1992), 32.
47. David M. Schneider and Raymond T. Smith, *Class Differences in American Kinship* (Ann Arbor: University of Michigan Press, 1978); Annette Lareau, *Unequal Childhoods: Class, Race, and Family Life* (Berkeley: University of California Press, 2003).
48. Teman, *Birthing a Mother.*
49. Amrita Pande, "'It May Be Her Egg but It's My Blood': Surrogates and Everyday Forms of Kinship in India," *Qualitative Sociology* 32, no. 4 (2009): 379–97. However, Rudrappa found that surrogates in Bangalore disclaim motherhood much like US surrogates, saying that the baby never was theirs; they belonged to someone else from the beginning. Sharmila Rudrappa, "India's Reproductive Assembly Line," *Contexts* 11, no. 2 (2012): 26–27.
50. E.g., Ragoné, *Surrogate Motherhood;* Hal B. Levine, "Gestational Surrogacy: Nature and Culture in Kinship," *Ethnology* 42 (2003): 173–85; Michael G. Peletz, "Kinship Studies in Late Twentieth-Century Anthropology," *Annual Review of Anthropology* 24 (1995): 343–72; Strathern, *Reproducing the Future*, 178.
51. Schneider (*American Kinship*) argued that sexual relations between husband and wife are the symbol of love (52).
52. Peletz, "Kinship Studies," 350.
53. Ibid., 351.
54. E-mail communication, 23 March 2010.
55. Teman, in *Birthing a Mother*, found the same for Israeli surrogates. However, "older and younger sisters" in the Indian context seems to indicate hierarchy, judging from data in Amrita Pande, *Wombs in Labor: Transnational Commercial Surrogacy in India* (New York: Columbia University Press, 2014). Rudrappa argued that Indian surrogates find sisterhood with fellow surrogates in the hostels where they are confined during the pregnancy in "India's Reproductive Assembly Line," 26.
56. Ragoné in *Surrogate Motherhood* and Roberts in "Examining Surrogacy Discourses" found this to be true. Teman documented that Israeli surrogates expected and cultivated a close connection with their intended mother rather than with the couple in *Birthing a Mother.*
57. Miranda, online surrogacy diary.
58. Ragoné, *Surrogate Motherhood*, 120–23.
59. Ilham Dillman, *Love and Human Separateness* (Oxford: Blackwell, 1987); Solomon, *About Love.*
60. Jenny, e-mail communication, 23 March 2010.
61. Jerome Bruner, *Making Stories: Law, Literature, Life* (Cambridge, MA: Harvard University Press, 2003), 17.

62. Ironically, this is the argument that critics have made against contractual enforcement.

63. A few surrogates pointed out that by reading the message boards IPs are able to figure out what surrogates want to hear and thus successfully deceive them.

64. Jenny, e-mail communication, 7 April 2010.

65. Clifford Geertz, *Interpretation of Cultures* (New York: Basic Books, 1973), 18.

66. Linda Layne argued in *Motherhood Lost. A Feminist Account of Pregnancy Loss in America,* (New York: Routledge, 2003) that medical advances promised women control over pregnancy and those who experience reproductive loss are confronted with a loss of control. The question of control is even more crucial for surrogates since surrogacy is a highly purposeful and self-consciously goal-oriented effort—the very metaphor of journey for surrogate pregnancy points to the surrogate's active role. Surrogate pregnancies never "happen"; they are always achieved.

67. A.E. Reading and J.F. Kerin, "Psychological Aspects of Providing Infertility Services," *Journal of Reproductive Medicine* 34 (1989): 861–71; Nancy E. Adler, Susan Keyes, and Patricia Robertson, "Psychological Issues in New Reproductive Technologies: Pregnancy-Inducing Technology and Diagnostic Screening," in *Women and New Reproductive Technologies: Medical, Psychological, Legal, and Ethical Dilemmas,* ed. J. Rodin and A. Collins (Hillsdale, NJ: Lawrence Erlbaum, 1991); Lauritzen, *Pursuing Parenthood.*

68. A "chemical pregnancy" is one in which the B-hCG pregnancy test is positive but the miscarriage happens before the gestational sac can be seen on ultrasound. A "blighted ovum" or "anembryonic pregnancy" is one in which the gestational sac is visible on ultrasound but a visible embryo does not develop. The word "miscarriage" is usually used for a pregnancy in which an embryo is visible on ultrasound.

69. Ragoné, *Surrogate Motherhood.*

70. Ava, e-mail communication, 2 May 2010. In this e-mail she also recounted the story of a fellow surrogate who gave birth to twins the same day Ava did and who did not post her story on SMO. That surrogate delivered six weeks early and experienced serious complications. Her IPs "alienated her completely. . . . The only thing that really pulled her through it (besides the medication . . .) was that she knew she has created two beautiful children."

71. William M. Reddy, *The Navigation of Feeling. A Framework for the History of Emotions* (Cambridge: Cambridge University Press, 2001), 323.

72. According to an SMO poll, only 13 of the 112 respondents said they did or planned to do only one surrogacy, mostly because of doctor's advice; 45 said two, 29 three, 25 said four or more.

73 Erving Goffman, *Relations in Public: Microstudies of the Public Order* (New York: Basic Books, 1971), 347.

74. Kapferer argued that "performance both expresses and creates what it represents." Bruce Kapferer, "Emotion and Feeling in Singhalese Healing Rites," *Social Analysis* 1 (1979): 153–54.

75. Erving Goffman, *The Presentation of Self in Everyday Life* (New York: Doubleday, 1959), 35.

76. Robert E. Park, *Race and Culture* (Glencoe, IL: Free Press, 1950), 294.

Chapter 3

CONTRACT

In the following, I first investigate the ways in which surrogates understand the contract and the issues that are contractually specified. Second, I document how relationships are negotiated through the contract. Third, I explore the lessons women drew from their experience and from SMO stories. Fourth, I describe and analyze surrogates' expectations and moral evaluations, given the lessons learned and the limits of the contract.

"contracts protect everyone"

Contracts, relationships, and contractual provisions

As we have seen, SMO-ers conceptualize surrogacy as an intimate and unique journey, but they also learn that the relationship with intended parents (IPs) may not always work out as expected. They realize that surrogate journeys call for not only sacrifices but also self-protections, and this conceptualization shapes their practical and moral evaluations. Keeping with the understanding that surrogacy is an intimate journey, women frequently reiterate that "if anyone tells you that there is an 'industry standard' in surrogacy that should be a heads-up for you to be wary because *nothing* is standard!" Yet they frequently compare contracts. Surrogates thus uphold the uniqueness of each journey while also gaining comparative insights into how to negotiate the contract.

Nevertheless, there is standardization; as much as the parties may negotiate directly, contracts are drawn up by increasingly specialized lawyers in the fairly new legal field of third-party reproduction. Intended parents and surrogates have their own legal counsel, and although IPs pay for all legal fees, surrogates choose their own lawyer, often based on recommendations from fellow surrogates.[1] Women increasingly know their rights and urge others to listen: "as far as her telling you to pick from 3 lawyers, it sounds to me like they are bulling you into that. You can pick ANY lawyer you want to look over your contract."

SMO discussions testify to the shared understanding that the contract is the first milestone of the journey. The financial and contractual side of surrogacy has become more visible and also more complicated with the rise of independent matching, in which the parties negotiate directly, and with new opportunities to negotiate with agencies. As independent arrangements multiplied and agency practices changed, contract discussions on SMO proliferated, testifying to an increasingly sophisticated grasp of legal logic.

But surrogates' frequent and involved discussions of the contract also reveal that such negotiations are uncomfortable because they represent calculation and lack of trust. Once in a while a newbie is so unwilling to negotiate that she starts medications without a contract. "I want so bad to be a great GS," wrote Jen. "I am cycling and there's been no talk of 'reimbursement.' . . . I realize that I have been doing too much in this relationship. (I was actually reading advice articles about dating to come to this conclusion—it is very much the same)." This post reveals the common dilemma of how to be a "great GS" without "doing too much" for the relationship and too little for oneself.

Yet Jen's post also exemplifies a behavior surrogates on SMO unanimously criticize. While wanting to be a great, caring, and sympathetic surrogate is admired, being uninformed and an easy target for potential mistreatment is never condoned. "I know you want to start your journey/adventure as a Surrogate but do it wisely so it will be an awesome one," advised Emily. Others agreed that Jen "made some bad choices" but that "it is not too late to make better ones." All the advice emphasized caution: "this is not how a good surrogacy relationship begins . . . contracts are essential before beginning the process." SMO-ers warn each other because informing and helping others is SMO's mission; it is also in their interest to collectively protect surrogacy as a practice by insisting on high standards of informed behavior.

Surrogacy contracts—increasingly detailed and often thirty to sixty pages long—specify a wide range of contingencies, responsibilities, and obligations beyond fees. Contracts most often include the number of times the parties will try to achieve pregnancy and, in gestational surrogacy, the number of pre-embryos to transfer. The parties increasingly frequently specify whether they are willing to selectively reduce (SR) in case of multifetal pregnancy or terminate a pregnancy in case of abnormalities. "Lifestyle prohibitions" are common as well, including various restrictions on travel, food and drink, medication, sex, and sometimes even hair coloring. Contracts always regulate the relinquishing of the baby to the IPs, often delineate who can be at the delivery, and sometimes set out the protocol for determining fault should the baby be born with "special needs."

A few IPs even wanted the surrogate not to post on SMO or any other support site, fearful that their privacy would be jeopardized. While SMO-ers may go along with IPs' requests that they eat organic food or not use Teflon pans or nail polish, they advise one another not to sign a contract that stipulates against the use of Internet support sites. They tend to find it offensive when IPs do not trust their surrogate to honor their privacy and that they would deprive her of the support she needs. To surrogates, these requests are often red flags that signal lack of both trust and empathy.

Contracts always specify the compensation and spell out the fee structure and payment schedule. Compensation is structured as either all inclusive (typically between $25,000 and $40,000)[2] or base compensation and extras (between $15,000 and $25,000, plus extra fees for various contingencies, e.g., invasive procedure, multiples, C-section, child care).[3] In an SMO poll, close to eighty percent of the 220 respondents preferred "base comp plus extras." Most surrogates favor this fee structure because it protects them and their families better and is less expensive for IPs given that most contingencies do not materialize. Negotiating a detailed list of "extras" is uncomfortable; it puts a price on pregnancy-related events and thus foregrounds the business aspect of surrogacy. Still, surrogates would agree with the following assessment: "I like the comfort of having a smaller fee with the extras 'just in case'. While I'd feel perfectly justified asking that high [45–50K] of an AI [all-inclusive] fee—I would feel bad b/c all those 'what-ifs' that I've covered in that fee might not happen."

In one of the many threads discussing fees, Henrietta spelled out her concerns, quite typical for those who contemplate all-inclusive compensation:[4]

I am a working professional and have two small children so if I was to do an all-inclusive arrangement I would have to take into consideration the potential for lost wages and child care. Only with those two things my fee would have to be more than 50K. I feel that that is still a gamble for me (just my salary is more than 50K) and also a gamble for my IP. . . . if I went all inclusive and then everything went well I would feel terrible taking all the extra money but I couldn't take the chance that something WOULD go wrong and then be left without any help.

Abigail explained a similar calculation: "'All-in' fee would be more than what my base comp would be. Only because it would cover every last 'what if' possible . . . (even though it may not happen)." In this post, Abigail describes a hypothetical situation ("would be"); she explains the logic of setting fees rather than her actual practice. Surrogates on SMO typically do not include "every last what if" because it would make the all-inclusive fee very expensive, and surrogates generally want to find the fairest solution for everyone: "I have a lot of things that I am hoping don't happen so the IPs do not have to spend the money on it. I obviously want to save the IPs as much money as possible, but also want to be fair to myself and to my family."

Thus, many surrogates who chose or agreed to an all-inclusive fee structure add a few essential extras to their all-in fees, for example, for child care, lost wages, and multiples, to be paid only when needed. This lowers the amount of the all-in compensation if all goes well, avoids having a long list of extras, and yet does not jeopardize the surrogate's financial security in case some of the what-ifs materialize.

Contracts also delineate the number of installments in which the surrogate is paid. Women prefer eight to ten equal payments, starting at either the first positive beta or at the first heartbeat.[5] On a pragmatic level, equal payments guarantee that women receive compensation for the duration of the pregnancy in case of miscarriage. But more importantly, such a schedule reflects the ongoing nature of pregnancy and everything it entails: "WHATEVER comp that you receive is for your pregnancy . . . the pain and suffering, loss of income from not being able to go to work, missed time with your kids, etc. NOT THE BABY!"

Surrogates warn everyone whose IPs want to pay at birth not to agree to a lump-sum payment: "the way this attorney is wording the contract is not the norm. . . . My contract pays 10 months of EQUAL payments. . . . I understand lowering your fee if you like your IPs . . . but I would NEVER accept . . . this contract." Marcia explained that this arrangement looks too much like "'baby selling'. You get your money when we get our baby." Lump-sum payment is uncomfortably similar to market exchange in which the relationship ends with monetary payment.

While lump-sum payments are problematic, the importance, indeed legitimacy, of compensation has long been established. "The amount of money in a surrogacy is not the point . . . it is the life that both parties together are creating. That being said money is the only way to compensate the time and sacrifice that will occur." When surrogates define the payment as compensation for "time and sacrifice" or, more commonly, for pain and suffering, they are not simply rejecting the stigma of baby selling or evading potential legal trouble. Rather, they are performing "relational work by means of monetary distinctions."[6] Through contractual and financial discussions, surrogates develop and negotiate the relationship with IPs and work out the definition of surrogacy.

More recently, surrogates have also been calling the compensation prebirth child support: "In my eyes and in my contract [compensation] is deemed prebirth child support because that is what it is. My IPs are paying me to carry, take care of and support their little ones until they are ready to take care of them. That is what child support is all about. It's to pay for expenses." Others point out the similarities between compensation and ex-husbands' child support payments. Implicitly, though, this comparison locates surrogacy in the intimate, private domain where people who created a child together do not always raise it together. By the same token, women also set "a boundary separating each relationship from others that resemble it in some regards" in this case, marriage on the one hand, and market transaction, on the other.[7]

Still, countless posts articulate discomfort with financial negotiations. Surrogates dislike the contract phase of the "journey"; they associate monetary negotiations with a cold and unfeeling economic rationality. Money in Western culture "signifies a sphere of economic relationships which are inherently impersonal, transitory, and calculating."[8] During negotiations women often worry about seeming greedy. Lori's dual concern about her contract and her IPs, for example, illuminates the dilemma many women face: "I don't want my IPs to feel like I am just trying to get their money, but I think some of these things [in the contract] aren't fair to me . . . but I don't want them to be upset about it." Even posts that advocate caution betray the conflict between "heart" and money: "It is not 'heartless' to care about protecting yourself and your family."

Instrumental and expressive contractual choices

In the earlier days of surrogacy, contract pregnancy had been problematized by various social critics who worried about commodification of women and babies.[9] However, there has been a noticeable
shift in the last decade or two in legal thinking toward pragmatic
considerations of predictability and protection.[10] Proponents consider the practice a mutually advantageous arrangement.[11] Intended
parents get a baby that is worth more than the payment to the
surrogate, while the money the surrogate receives is more than
the risks she takes.[12] Relying on the same logic, Richard Epstein
maintained that voluntary exchange "promotes human welfare"
even if some exchange is offensive to some people.[13] He claimed
that enforceable contracts are sufficient to guarantee good outcomes
between rational actors. "The terms and conditions of the relationship can be fully explained . . . to the potential surrogate."[14]

But most SMO discussions reveal a somewhat different lived
experience in which risks are neither fully known nor fully know-
able. Sarah was responding to a discussion about an "expenses only,"
that is, uncompensated surrogacy, but her story is not uncommon,
and her advice to others is quite typical:

> I went into my first surrogacy thinking the exact same way as many
> surros. I don't want this to be about money so my "fee" was on the
> small end. Well guess what . . . I transferred two embies and both
> took. I ended up on bedrest from 22 two weeks on. Then I went
> into the hospital at 30 weeks with preeclampsia and was delivered
> by emergency c-section. Because I had preeclampsia . . . I bled out
> and almost lost my uterus. . . . I did this from the bottom of my
> heart but how can someone who has never done a surrogacy truly
> know what's going to happen. my sons were both full term vaginal
> births with no complications. You cannot predict what is going to
> happen . . . my family had to give up their time and energy and they
> did not have their mom for almost 4 months. I feel for these couples
> who cannot have children otherwise I wouldn't have done it. But
> you have to look out for your OWN family first and foremost. NOT
> the IPs. I didn't do that and my family sacrificed. . . . I would do it all
> over again in a second but when deciding what type of compensation
> you want think long and hard about EVERYONE involved.

Sarah's call for thinking "long and hard" about compensation
sounds more like a strategy to avoid loss rather than to "rationally
maximize" expected gain, which is the main premise of contract
law.[15] Underlying this premise are the social propositions that

the parties to the contract are the best judges of their own utility, that they "normally reveal their determination of utility in their promises," that contractual promises are deliberatively made "for personal gain," and that contract bargaining enables the parties to "plan their future conduct reliably."[16] Conventional contract theory assumes that rational people who enter into a contractual relationship are making an instrumental selection from alternative future options and that these options are comparable. But these definitions of contract and benefit are not helpful for understanding the position surrogates take.

SMO posts indicate that surrogates know that no matter how well informed they are, they cannot "plan their future conduct reliably" or "rationally maximize" their expected utility.[17] Countless threads attest to surrogates' efforts to reconcile helping IPs with reasonable self-protection. "The first step is to get the contract in place. . . . Make sure you are all on the same page each step of the way, communicate frequently . . . don't take shortcuts or push the proper procedure off just because you're anxious to help another family out." However, repeated calls for self-protection indicate that surrogates know they may get too caught up in their effort to "make dreams come true."

Gillian Hadfield questioned the universal applicability of the conventional conceptualization of contract and proposed that choices have to do with valuation, which is not simply quantitative but also qualitative.[18] Our choices are not merely instrumental; they express and construct who we are.[19]

> An expressive choice to enter into a contract may spring not from an assessment of the value of future consequences, but rather from a person's judgment that, in the present moment, signing a given contract adequately expresses her valuation of the situation, another person, or herself . . . choice may have been *fundamentally* [italics in original] an expression of her valuation of the present circumstances and not an expression of her consequential assessment of future options.[20]

By all accounts, SMO-ers value children and family; the decision to become a surrogate is greatly influenced by stories of infertility. Imagination plays a role here; most surrogates confess to not having personally experienced this painful situation.[21] To familiarize themselves with it, SMO-ers are happy to read accounts and watch videos of infertility stories and stories of years of treatment, failure, and heartache. Confronted with the problem of infertility, surrogates respond in ways that express what they proudly call their "caring and compassionate" nature. "How could anyone hear the stories I've heard and not be moved to action??! But I think it does take a unique and special personality," wrote Tasha. This formulation nicely captures the way surrogates understand their own significance: although stories of infertility should move people to action, only special women take up the challenge. Entering into a surrogacy contract expresses women's valuation of babies and family *and* their expectations to be valued for helping to create them.

Determination to help notwithstanding, surrogates often emphasize the importance of being level-headed about contract negotiations even as they are excited to embark on a "wonderful journey." Given pervasive dichotomous understandings of emotions and rationality,[22] whenever surrogates highlight empathy as the basis of their ethical outlook, they also go to great lengths to affirm their commitment to rational conduct. They do not want to appear emotionally driven and irrational. "Contracts protect everyone. . . . use your head, not just your heart," is the oft-repeated advice that SMO-ers do not always follow. Rationality is central to contractual agreements. However, surrogates' emphasis on rationality and reliability achieves more than signaling assurance that they will live up to the terms of the contract and not "keep the baby."[23] Surrogates articulate the morality of giving but in many ways also embrace the culturally compelling and widely shared morality of rational action.[24] In a post about the distinguishing traits of a good surrogate, women added knowledge of the process and being proactive to a list that contained compassion, sympathy, care, understanding, and honesty.

My argument about surrogates' contractual decisions has less to do with individual personality traits or attitudes and more to do with collective interpretive processes that create meaning and inform behavior. Lay understandings of law are "formed within and changed by social action."[25] SMO discussions constitute social action and interaction that construct and shape meanings. Collective interpretive communications on SMO generate, promote, and reward certain understandings of the contract and certain norms of valuation.

"business and the wonderful bond"

Negotiating relationships

"It does sound harsh, but this is a business transaction to a point. . . . At times it can be hard to separate the two (business and the wonderful bond that grows), but you have to or that is when things can go haywire." This formulation is quite typical and sheds light on surrogates' notion that the "business of surrogacy" is the sound basis from which a good relationship grows and that getting the details right is a necessary, although by no means sufficient, condition of a "wonderful bond." By using the verb "to separate," this surrogate conveyed the idea that business and personal relationship are entwined in surrogacy.

Joanna went further in highlighting the relational aspect of contracts; she explained that even though contracts are not always legally recognized, "the process of discussing the contract helps set the ground rules and expectations for the journey and that is very important. Discussing contract items tends to bring out the worst in people, so it is a good way to see how people react to stress."[26] Her explanation highlights the shared SMO contention that contract negotiations have predictive value for the personal relationship with IPs.

Ava pointed out that attention to detail is not a sign of distrust but a way to guarantee better outcomes:

> Anytime you hear of something going wrong in surrogacy, it is because something was missed in the contract, or there wasn't a contract at all. For me, it was so vital that we include everything. It wasn't that I didn't trust my IPs. I absolutely did and still do. You just never know. It's kind of like no one goes into a marriage with the intentions of getting divorced. But it happens.[27]

Ava emphasizes the importance of the contract precisely because she, much like others on SMO, sees the relationship with her IPs as a personal one. Like many other surrogates, she compares surrogacy to marriage; and in intimate, personal relationships, unplanned things can "happen." Her response also points to the role SMO stories play in shaping expectations and attitudes and in inculcating responsibility for one's journey.

But "the business of surrogacy" means more for surrogates than merely careful attention to detail. Negotiations are indicative of the rapport surrogates hope to have: "it's how you all handle the negotiations which will clue you in on your future relationship and communications." This understanding of the contract further illuminates why surrogates worry so much not to seem "money hungry."[28] It is during contract discussions that surrogates negotiate the personal relationship with their IPs, establish themselves as sympathetic and giving women, and signal that they expect sympathy and care in return.

Elizabeth was hesitant to ask for a fee for potential complications, fearful that her "perfect couple" would think she cared only about money. Others reminded her, "If they were so perfect they would understand your concerns and help." No response referenced conventional contractual protection; rather, women spoke of concern, care, and help. Libby pointed out that if IPs "truly care about" the surrogate, they accommodate her, as long as her requests are reasonable. Surrogates see negotiations as a litmus test of character and compatibility, rather than simply a means to a fair contract.

But even when qualities like care and valuation are deemed non-reducible to quantity, they are negotiated through financial dealings. Ann, who started medication without a finalized contract in order to "speed up" the process, wanted to include a fee for bed rest, but her IM disagreed because Ann only worked part time. Lilly's was one of the many sympathetic responses; she also started medication before the contract was signed. She offered her story as an example to follow. Lilly's couple did not agree to the bed rest fee either, and she "walked away" because "if they couldn't see me as more than a uterus, then it wasn't going to happen. They needed to realize that . . . the fact that I was going to carry their baby couldn't get in the way of my family's well-being." Lilly's story reveals that practical considerations are pregnant with symbolic meanings: money covers potential income loss and also stands for the concern and respect surrogates want for themselves and their family.

Contractual sacrifices

Surrogates insist they should never have to suffer the consequences of lost wages and child care costs, but even here we see some variation in practice. For example, many surrogates use vacation days, sick days, and short-term disability to cover days they had to take off for appointments or other pregnancy-related issues to save money for IPs. Helping IPs to save money is a way of expressing empathy and care. However, caring for IPs competes with protecting surrogates' and their family's interest. Surrogates can easily find themselves in a situation where helping their IPs may hurt their own family: "I certainly don't want to nickel and dime my IPs, but at the same time I would hate to use up all my time [sick leave and vacation] for my family with a pregnancy for someone else." The complicating factor is that surrogates often need to make decisions in the present without information about the future; present concerns are frequently more pressing than future what-ifs.

At the time of contract negotiations, surrogates and IPs are often concerned that reimbursement for lost wages may add up to be very expensive, especially with multifetal pregnancies and bed rest. Having disability insurance lowers the amount IPs have to pay and makes it easier for them to agree to covering lost wages during contract negotiations. However, many workplaces mandate that employees use all their paid time off (PTO) before they can use short-term disability, as this surrogate did:[29] "My job does have disability benefits that will cover me for any bedrest time—I have to use all my PTO first, then disability will kick in. It's not 100% (I don't know the exact %), so my contract states that my IPs will cover any of my salary above and beyond disability."

Because of this workplace policy, some women had used up all their paid time off for surrogacy-related appointments or ailments in order to be able to use their disability coverage and save IPs money. They discovered later, when their own children became ill, that they had to take unpaid leave. They warn others on SMO not to repeat their mistake: "Do not short yourself or your family, no one wants to take advantage of their IPs but you do not want to put your own family at financial risk when you are helping someone else create a family or add to it."

Fees for invasive procedures, multiples, and C-sections are also very common and offer financial protection for the surrogate and her family. Even though these contingencies are often interrelated, they represent different hardships; for example, carrying multiples may be a harder pregnancy and often leads to Cesarean delivery, the C-section makes recovery longer and is thus an additional hardship that surrogates usually want to be compensated for. However, in the spirit of fairness, some women consider it unreasonable to charge a C-section fee if the surrogate had previous Cesareans and is likely to deliver that way again. Others insist that C-section fees are necessary no matter what: "it covers the childcare/recover needs/lost wages from the procedure."

Similarly, maternity clothes allowance sometimes gives rise to disagreements on the boards. Some argue that repeat surrogates who had already accumulated a pregnancy wardrobe should charge less or not at all for maternity clothes. An experienced surrogate posted the following: "I still have tons of maternity clothes that fit just fine, so I prefer to stick w/those, and I don't mind shopping for maternity clothes at garage sales, thrift stores, etc." However, there are women who report spending more than the allowance without asking for reimbursement. "Interesting that the vast majority of surros spend out of pocket $ for mat[ernity] clothes," commented an old-timer. The reasons behind this are spelled out in the following: "Personally I feel like during that 9 months I would have purchased new clothing anyway, so if I add some to the pot that is fine. I probably spend $300 to $400 each 6 months on clothes anyway, so I don't mind adding that amount to the maternity allowance."

Another contentious topic is retainers, that is, payment to retain the surrogate in case IPs cannot start right away. Many women question the legitimacy of such payments. As Wanda wrote, "Unless you are doing this for the financial gain . . . do you need to be paid for building a relationship with your IPs?" Jeanne agreed; if surrogates say "'they're the perfect IPs I just love them' . . . then isn't that enough retainer?" Some others think retainers guarantee that the IPs "have serious intentions." Most surrogates are either against a retainer fee or consider it advance payment, designed to guarantee commitment, rather than an extra fee.

The question of including "lost reproductive organ fees" in the contract also stirred a few heated debates. One camp insisted that surrogates should know full well the potential risks of pregnancy and birth and not charge extras for them. "This is not a way for me to make money, so it's not like a loss that would impact my lifestyle, like a painter who loses their arms, or a roofer who loses their legs." This line of argument holds that not being able to carry again cannot be measured in monetary terms. Thus loss of reproductive ability is not akin to work-related injuries and should not be compensated. Arguing against these fees is tantamount to emphasizing the difference between market work and surrogacy.

Dissenting surrogates agree with this premise but explain that loss of reproductive ability would entail health consequences such as surgeries, recovery periods, and medications that are indeed measurable in dollars. "Losing some type of reproductive organ after birth implies some kind of complication to me. This fee . . . covers the complication. IE; time off of work, childcare, housekeeping, recovery, etc. I do not 'do this for money' either. If I am out of commission, my family suffers financially. THEY always need to be taken care of."

In these threads women contest and negotiate not only what fees to include in the contract but also the symbolic meaning of surrogacy and the reasonable scope of sacrifice. Whether they charge fees for C-section or reproductive organ loss or not, women assert that creating families is the ultimate goal and it is worth the sacrifice, but one's own family deserves to be protected. "Making sure surrogacy does not cost your family is not greedy." Marianna put it this way: "how can I go and put my family at risk in that way when we aren't rich? It would be sooo unfair to my own babies if I were in the hospital for weeks, they were in full time daycare, and we went broke, risked losing our own home etc. . . . for somebody I barely know."

Surrogates thus establish equality between the value of the family they help create and that of their own. Equality becomes an issue not only because IPs are typically more affluent than surrogates but also because surrogates themselves emphasize how much the babies they gestate for their IPs are wanted and precious life. But no matter how precious these yearned-for babies are, or how much money it takes to create them, they are not more valuable than the surrogate's own children and creating them should not jeopardize the well-being of the surrogates' family.

"I learned my lesson well"

Giving and getting

Keeping the interest of one's family in mind is a recurrent theme precisely because surrogates tend to get caught up in "making people's dream come true"; they attribute this to their "natural inclination to give." Natalie, whose first IPs failed to pay more than a thousand dollars in pregnancy-related medical bills after she gave birth to triplets, vowed "to not give sooo much of myself," the second time around. Other women make similar resolutions: "My promise to myself and others is that I will take every reasonable step to protect myself this time around. . . . I have that little character flaw that so many of us women have. . . . I give too much."

However, discussions reveal that the problem is not simply "giving too much." Voluntary and informed giving is considered a virtue; being "too giving" means giving more than one had intended to. There are surrogates who did not get any compensation when their pregnancy ended in miscarriage because of the way the contract was worded. Others failed to receive a fee for some invasive procedure because it was not specified in the contract or ended up with a net loss after being put on bed rest because there was a cap on lost wages or childcare. "I wish I could warn every single NEW surrogate please please please be careful. Cover all the bases. I have lost so much money. I have almost lost my job . . . all for providing someone else a miracle," wrote Eve, thirty-two weeks pregnant with twins. "This will answer the question . . . about why comp was raised the second time. It's all about learning," concluded a three-time surrogate.

Kathy's story reveals a similar learning curve. Initially, she thought that she and her IPs "were perfect for each other." She lowered her compensation "out of love" and left things they verbally agreed upon out of the contract so as not to "hurt their feelings" by being too focused on "having it in writing." But things "went horribly wrong . . . in the end our magical journey was nothing more than a business deal. We were to follow our contract exactly, leaving some of my pregnancy expenses to come out of my already low comp." But Kathy did not blame her IPs. "It was my fault! I learned my lesson well! Next time I will not be lowering my comp, and I will know exactly what needs to be in my contract to cover my family, not my IPs'."

Surrogates clearly learn from their past mistakes, and from other women's. SMO data indicate that experienced surrogates are more likely to learn from both. In threads about contract issues women swap stories about what went wrong; the initial post thus gives rise to stories and discussions about a range of omissions and ambiguities in contracts that hurt surrogates. Learning seems to accelerate once a surrogate has her own bad experience. Wendy carried triplets, born just short of twenty-eight weeks:

> I understand that should the babies not make it the surro may not receive comp, but my IPs went home with 3 babies, and because the contract was worded a certain way, I received less than 50% of my total comp (triplets). I even received less than the agreed upon comp for a singleton. The journey was not about the money, but I lost my job. . . . Throw in there the hospital stay, the bedrest, etc. . . . After this happened to me I did a lot of hindsight research.

Ashley also started to pay more serious attention to what other surrogates were saying after she paid hundreds of dollars for medical bills. "I had so many surrogates, and even a few IPs, telling me what a crock my contract was but didn't know until it was too late and I didn't think anything would go wrong."

Newbies tend to be less circumspect, and often more trusting, as the above posts show. "I didn't think anything would go wrong" is a recurrent phrase in surrogates' narratives. For those who read SMO posts, however, it has become increasingly hard to disregard advice that explicitly confronts this attitude: "The most important thing . . . is to forget all about your feelings for your IPs when you're going over your contract. Listen to what experienced surrogates tell you when they are trying to give you advice. And don't ever think that 'it'll never happen to me', because that's when it does."

And increasingly, newbies do listen. Doreen, for example, felt a little "rushed" but was determined "to take whatever time I need to get this exactly how I need it to be. Of course my lawyer will be examining it, but I want to know exactly what you felt was most important or you wish you had included in your contract." One of the many responses was from Cindy, another newbie: "While I was reading here and getting ready to even see a contract . . . I took notes from every contract thread that was started." Cindy then posted a long list of the essential provisions she had gleaned from her research. Only some of these essentials are financial issues, as I will discuss later in this chapter.

There are unmistakable signs of learning; SMO discussions have become more sophisticated and more detailed. Many more newbies ask for advice about contractual provisions, indicating increased interest and attentiveness to details. This has to do with surrogates' ability to negotiate even when they work with an agency, let alone in independent arrangements. If cautionary statements like the following are not new, they have become more frequent: "I changed 5 pages in my contract the first time around! I wanted to make sure my family is covered! Your family should never have to suffer a minute cause you are helping another become a family!" New surrogates on SMO consciously want to learn from other women's stories and advice: "I just got the 1st draft of our contract and I am afraid I am missing something. I am so new to this and I don't want to just accept the 'standard issue' contract the agency sends to everyone. If you had to do it all over again what would you do differently?" posted Alinda, who was then commended for doing her homework. SMO-ers applaud surrogates who negotiate carefully and are unkind to those who rush into signing a contract.

SMO discussions clearly indicate that women have access to information and routinely ask questions and compare notes about contracts. They increasingly regard it as a deal breaker when IPs want to cap coverage for lost wages or childcare costs, since these are the two biggest financial risk factors. The most discussed non-financial topics are the number of pre-embryos to transfer, selective reduction, and termination. There has been a noticeable change from the early 2000s as women have become more aware of the potential dangers of multifetal pregnancy and of the physical and emotional repercussions of selective reduction and termination. Yet women want to balance protecting themselves with benefitting their IPs.

Pressures

In practice, this balancing act is very hard, especially when IPs seem desperate to have a baby, which they most often do, even when they already have children. Leah's couple wanted her to sign a contract that gave her no say in how many pre-embryos to transfer. Because of her IM's advanced age and history of heart-break, Leah explained, she wanted to do everything in her power to maximize the chances of pregnancy and left the decision to the IPs. In spite of advice from fellow surrogates who first warned, then criticized her, she signed the contract, asserting that she was "an educated woman who did her research." Her IPs took the reproductive endocrinologist's advice, and four pre-embryos were transferred into Leah's uterus. Leah's case may be somewhat extreme; it is not common to sign such a contract. However, as many threads testify, balancing self-protection with respecting IPs' wishes is not easy, given IPs' and surrogates' eagerness to achieve pregnancy, the high cost of repeated IVF procedures, and the time it takes to do repeated cycles.

A good example of a discussion of such a balancing act is when Ginger, a new surrogate whose IPs had twins, asked for advice on whether to transfer three pre-embryos:

> We transferred two . . . and ended up with a chemical pregnancy. My IPs have one straw left with three embryos in it. . . . I was/am only willing to transfer 2. (I have four kids under 6) and if I had to go on bedrest and put my kids in daycare, and put all that stress on my husband, I could never forgive myself. But there is still a part of me that wonders if I did transfer three, what are my chances of triplets. I REALLY want this to work for them, and they only have three left. Would you guys ever transfer three, or is this a classic "desperate rookie" mistake?[30]

Fellow surrogates advised against transferring three: "in your situation [i.e., good embryo quality] no I don't think I would transfer 3.

I know negatives REALLY suck and you want this to work, just remember you have to make these sorts of decisions with your head more than your heart, as hard as that is sometimes!!" All responses cautioned her but also acknowledged Ginger's feelings: "I would not transfer three, though I do understand the feeling of wanting to do anything to help. The risk of triplets is too great—to me, to the babies, to IPs, to my family." Ginger reported back:

> Thank you for sharing all of this information with me. I am going to stick to my guns and stay with only transferring 2. . . . My IM wants me to consider three, I have said two, but she keeps lightly suggesting it. Thank goodness for contracts! But it does have me second guessing my plans. . . . But, I need to remember my family first, and then theirs.☺ . . . My IM knows the risks of triplets, but I just think she is desperate for twins since this is her last straw and her last chance. Sheesh, talk about pressure.☻

A few days later Ginger posted again, "totally not sure what to do":

> I just talked to the RE yesterday and explained the situation to her and she said that she felt very comfortable transferring the 3 day embryos. She . . . said that the chance of triplets is less than 5%. My IPs originally had 12 embryos to start they are down to the last three, out of the nine that have been transferred only 2 have resulted in live pregnancies, the twins. . . . I am so torn on what to do. Part of me just wants to do all three and let the good Lord decide what He wants me to have, and another part of me is so scared of triplets. My husband is totally on board for doing all three.

SMO-ers still considered it too risky and called attention to the importance of rational thinking. Strikingly, no one questioned why IPs who already have twins would be so "desparete for twins" that they would pressure their surrogate to agree to transferring more than she wants to: "I understand that they're feeling desperate, which leads to emotions taking over, but some serious and rational thought needs to be put into this decision, by everyone. Throwing more embryos in doesn't increase the chance of success by much, but it dramatically increases the odds of multiples." Everyone advised her against transferring all three embryos, and all responses advocated rational thinking, reminding her that the goal is "to birth a live healthy baby."

All the advice to the contrary notwithstanding, women noticed Ginger's increasing willingness to accommodate her IPs: "you sound like you talked yourself into doing what your IPs want. I hope that turns out in your best interest, and your family. I know it's hard to stand up against the pressure, been there and caved myself. But I learned one heck of a lesson, that hurt me and my family. I hope you don't regret anything." But Ginger thought about her decision differently:

> I wouldn't say I have talked myself into what the IPs want. . . . More like I have re-evaluated the situation, found out some important facts on the embryo quality and egg donor, taken the advice of the doctor, and this being my IPs' last three embryos am willing to take the "less than 2% chance of triplets. I was just asking for insight on transferring two versus three embryos from surrogates on this board who have been around the block a time or two. I have since learned that there is no magic number and every surrogate has to make that personal decision on her own. I have decided that my number for this next transfer is going to be three based on facts, NOT on emotion.

It is interesting to note that even though donor eggs were involved in this surrogacy and the IPs already had twins, neither Ginger nor anyone else asked why this was considered the IPs' "last chance." Surrogates who advocate rational thinking do not question the rhetoric of "last chance" or "IPs' desperation." However, when surrogates evaluate other surrogates' decisions, rationality is highly rated on the boards. Thus, Ginger framed her change of heart as a rational and informed decision rather than an emotional one.

Encountering pressure after signing the contract is not rare, and there were other surrogates who changed their mind at the time of the transfer much like Ginger did. Thinking about a case of quadruple pregnancy that captured SMO-ers attention in 2007, Alyson invited fellow surrogates to discuss transfer practices:

> In my contract, it says we would not transfer more than 2 embryos. I never wanted to transfer more embryos. However, on transfer day, our embryos were pretty poor in quality and had we had more . . . and had my IM asked me to, I probably would have transferred more. As a surrogate, I know that I would have felt a ton of pressure. We are already under a ton of stress, knowing that we are our IPs only shot at a baby and I know that I would have had a hard time putting my foot down. . . . it just makes me wonder how many surrogates REALLY agree to more than they would like to. Also, who's responsible? I guess I think if the surro agrees, then she has to take the consequences and is responsible for her actions, but do the IPs and the RE have any responsibility to the surrogate?

Responses indicate that quite a few surrogates transferred more than they had contractually agreed to:

> My contract says 2 or we can transfer more upon REs recommendation. My IM has been through a lot and our 1st cycle ended with NO embryos. . . . After that my husband and I discussed it and we told our IPs we would be willing to transfer as many as they wanted to transfer and the RE would allow. We only had three that made it to transfer and we transferred all of them.

The desire to make the IPs parents often prevails over the contractual agreement. After the RE's recommendation, Sharon disregarded her contract and agreed to transferring four the first time and six the second time: "My IM had a long journey with failed attempts, miscarriage (1st and 2nd trimester) and I really wanted to be 'the one' to help her become a mom. I was willing and fully accepting the possibility of carrying 3. We were given such a low chance of just ONE sticking." SMO-ers maintain that if the surrogate consents to transferring as many as the IPs and the RE decide, she is responsible for the outcome.

> My 1st transfer we transferred 4. The quality wasn't that great, and if all 4 took, we were reducing down to twins. We all went into it with eyes wide open.
>
> 2nd transfer we did 3. Quality again wasn't good. We would have reduced down to twins. Yes I agree if you don't want to reduce, only transfer what you are willing to carry. But then you also need to take into consideration what the doctor says about the quality and IPs' finances. But if we, as carriers, agree to it then we also have to own up to the responsibility.

However, surrogates increasingly vehemently condemn selective reduction as a terrible way "to correct mistakes." Opposition to selective reduction is the crystallization of countless debates and stories of regret: "We want to create life, not take life." Women increasingly urge newbies to think through where they stand on selective reduction and make this stance clear in contractual terms. SMO-ers are not kind to fellow surrogates who chose to close their eyes rather than confront the possibility that their couple could think about these issue differently. Neither are they sympathetic to women who agree to selective reduction, especially after the many cautionary stories and passionate discussions on the boards. Julia, a three-time surrogate, warned a newbie who was about to sign a contract. The IPs wanted to transfer two pre-embryos and to reduce to a singleton in case of twin pregnancy.

You also need to consider that a good portion of doctors won't reduce twin to singleton and you may have to travel to do the procedure. I would run from this situation. . . . We were on our third cycle. We had previously transferred 3 with no viable pregnancy. . . . When we were on the brink of transfer my IPs decided that they couldn't do twins. I made the decision to transfer two knowing I would have to reduce one. I was naive. I thought there was little chance of twins. Our odds were really low. . . . I thought the pain of letting my IPs walk away without the baby they wanted so badly would be worse than a reduction. Talk about ridiculous! I know that would have hurt as well but nowhere near the pain of a reduction. We were about 13 weeks. I encourage you to look up ultrasound pictures of 12 and 13 week fetuses. They already look like little babies. . . . They use an ultrasound to guide a needle into the baby's heart and inject poison into it and watch it until it stops beating. I will never be the same care free person. . . . My thought process is that I gave that baby life and I took it away because he wasn't wanted. It kills me.

The heartache over the reduction was not the only hardship Julia had. She experienced serious complications from the procedure and was on bed rest for fourteen weeks, most of it in the hospital. She missed her children's graduations, and she lost her job as a consequence. She delivered at thirty weeks.

Kate's post is a good indication of SMO hostility to selective reduction, even among women who are pro-choice:

The idea of reducing for convenience makes me physically ill. Make no mistake, I am 110% pro-choice, accidents happen and I don't think anyone should have to pay for them for the rest of their lives. . . . But in surrogacy (and IVF) there are no accidents and we have HOM [higher-order multiples] control from the very start. Those embryos were purposely transferred, if your IPs absolutely only want one, ONLY TRANSFER ONE.

Surrogates have become very vocal about the need to carefully specify in the contract not only whether they agree to selective reduction but also the conditions or abnormalities for which they are willing to terminate a pregnancy:

I want this thread to be about how important it is to have your contract worded appropriately. . . . As far as those that agree to s/r or termination, contracts need to be very specific unless you are willing to go along with anything. I know a lot of surros that agree to s/r or termination have very specific ideas of when, how, and why they would agree to it. If they don't have that in the contract they leave themselves open to issues if the IPs want to terminate for something like a club foot or cleft palate. . . . What if they want to terminate because they find out it's not the gender they wanted? . . . Perhaps surros need to state what they WILL NOT terminate or reduce for along with what they will. If someone has a contract that is spelled out very specifically about how they will or won't terminate perhaps they could share here how it's written in hopes of helping out someone else down the road.

Increasingly, discussions focus on the surrogate's responsibility to clarify her views before contract negotiations precisely because it is her body that is gestating the IPs' baby:

> I often see, especially with first time surrogates, the mentality of "their babies their decision." I was one of those people! I think it's vitally important to balance that with the reality that it is your body and you will live with the physical and emotional repercussions for life. . . . I believe on hot topics like this you should definitely have it spelled out very clear and concise. . . . in the heat and emotion of a situation you cannot make a clear decision on in the moment.

Experienced surrogates emphasize how important it is not to compromise: "it's important to know where you stand on the issue and match with like-minded IPs."

Old-timers understand other surrogates' decisions better and may be more tolerant but not necessarily more yielding: "I can see why people make the decision now, but I still know it is not the right decision for me." Even when they hold uncompromising views, most surrogates reassure others that they are not judging anyone: "I will not terminate for any reason (except if my own life is in danger). I believe in God's sovereignty. I always have been pro-life and I always be. While I may not condone or agree with the choices others make, I am not judgmental. Only they will have to live with the consequences of the choices they make."

Being against termination of any sort may make it harder to match, some women say, but it is crucial to be "on the same page with IPs." The more they read stories in which surrogates who hoped that "it wouldn't happen to them" were confronted with decisions about termination, the more they see the necessity for clarifying these issues with prospective IPs:

> I've always been pro-life for myself, but when I first started researching surrogacy I felt like it wasn't my baby, so I wouldn't have a say. Reading . . . of GS who dealt with SR for HOM and one for Downs

had me in tears—I would have that on my conscience for the rest of my life. It is definitely one of the more unpleasant things to discuss with new IPs, but very necessary.

The view that 'it's not my baby", that babies always belong to the IPs, holds that the "IPs have the ultimate right in deciding what is best for their situation. I would never take that decision away from them." "I, for one, completely separate myself from my GS pregnancies and completely see them as not my own, but my IFs' pregnancy, just with a little of my help added in. Therefore, how in the world could **I** tell **THEM** how to make a decision regarding something that will affect *them* their entire life?" Not all surrogates are able to separate themselves from the pregnancy this way even when they easily separate pregnancy from motherhood. SMO-ers have a few distinctively different solutions to the two separations surrogacy requires them to make: gestation and parenthood, on the one hand, and body and self, on the other.

Elly Teman's findings about Israeli surrogates' "body map" point to consistent identifications of certain body parts and not others with the self. Wombs were not viewed as intimately connected to the person; wombs can carry a baby without personally involving the surrogate in the pregnancy.[31] US surrogates use many of the same metaphors as their Israeli counterparts—babysitter, oven, incubator—indicating that they easily separate womb/gestation and self/parenthood. But when they contemplate selective reduction and termination, US surrogates tend to see their wombs as part of the self, even as they do not consider themselves the parent of the baby they carry. In these situations the effort to separate the pregnant body from the empathetic self that values life gives rise to troubling questions. If surrogates endure hardship to give couples babies, how can they "take life" that is viable just because IPs want fewer or more perfect babies? How can IPs be both "desperate" and selective? And if desperation and selective practices coexists, what are the implications for surrogates?

Surrogate morality

Numerous discussions take up these issues, and SMO consensus stops short of embracing the "it is their baby; it is their decision" stance, even though some women still hold this view. Much more common is the following position, the outcome of years of debates that consider both the IPs' sovereign parenthood and surrogates' moral world view, informed and shaped by stories of heartache and remorse:

Who am I to decide what someone should or shouldn't have to go through. On the other hand, I just don't know how I would deal with being a part of the choice if the time came. So, I think it is best for me to look for like-minded IPs. I respect those SMs who can go forward and respect the IPs wishes no matter what, but I don't think I could be one of them.

Surrogates often cannot separate body and self as easily as they uncouple gestation and parenthood. The solution emerged from the many selective reduction/termination threads: "[Termination] should be WELL thought about BEFORE you find yourself in that situation." "I just want other surros to please, PLEASE know that this can happen to you and make sure your contract reflects not only how you *think* you **FEEL** at the time of signing, but also the way you will **ACT** if it ever happens to you." Through discussions, surrogates develop a sense of responsibility that may be at odds with contractual specifications:

> I don't understand how a piece of paper (contract), or wishes of IPs (termination), could come before the life of a child. Where is our priority as a surrogate? Is it to IPs only? Or to IPs, and the child second? . . . Maybe I'm wrong in the matter, but the safety of the child comes first, and IPs second with me. That child entrusted his life to me when choosing to take hold and grow, and I will never allow someone to go in and end that life. That would be my choice to allow that to happen, breaking my promise to that baby to keep him safe, most especially for the reason of, "You're not perfect, and therefore not wanted." Painful to the IPs? Of course. . . . Painful to the surro? Absolutely. So then is the growing baby just an object whose life doesn't matter, especially if the biological parents say, "terminate"? . . . Where does our responsibility lie to that child, as a surrogate?

These are very troubling questions, and surrogates would love to believe that IPs only terminate for extremely serious abnormalities: "Most likely if the IPs do decide to terminate, it isn't because the babies' eye color is wrong, or some minor problem. It is something huge." Yet what is a "huge problem" to some IPs (e.g., Down syndrome, dwarfism) does not seem huge to many surrogates, who would rather find adoptive parents than terminate:

> It seems common for IPs to feel that if they can't raise the child their surro is carrying, for whatever reason (usually Down's, etc.) then they will choose to abort and don't feel comfortable signing over rights so that their surro can raise the child or could find a home

that would like to adopt the child. I can understand why as IPs you may feel unable to raise this child, but why not allow the surrogate to raise or adopt out? Why is termination the only option when there IS another home that would want the baby?

The most discussed and controversial condition for termination is Down syndrome. Many surrogates do not understand why IPs want to terminate such an "otherwise healthy" pregnancy, even when they respect IPs' decision of not wanting to raise such a child. In an SMO poll 70 of the 132 respondents said they would terminate for Down syndrome at the IPs' request, while the rest said that they would not. It is not only surrogates who highlight the importance of being "on the same page" about these issues with IPs. In one contentious thread Christina, an IM, urged fellow IPs to only match with surrogates who share their views on termination:

> if any woman would terminate for any reason why isn't she asked to give up her child for adoption? She isn't because she is seen as its mother. Why are we considered by a different standard? Once my child is conceived it is my child. My heart and soul know no difference of where the baby is carried. I am its parent and I would not ever adopt out my child to anyone. . . . I highly recommend any surro who is not okay with s/r or termination not agree to it. It would be a compromise of one's soul and not worth the personal damage it could forever cause. I strongly recommend to all IPs regardless of their personal position on S/R and Termination to make it their choice by working with a surrogate who will allow them the parental decision.

This post and others like it put surrogates in a somewhat uncomfortable position. They very much agree that the babies they carry belong to the IPs; they have no problem separating gestation from parenthood. At the same time SMO-ers also strongly believe that every life is precious and that surrogacy means creating life:

> To assume the child will face a lifetime of pain isn't really fair. YES there are the ones who do and die early or are never able to lead independent lives. But at the same time, there are a lot who can. Why not celebrate the time you do have with your child, be it 2 years or 20 years?

Olivia's response went a little too far and rattled quite a few IMs and surrogates:

> If a child can have a chance at life, I am all for it. I think saying "Either I get to raise a perfect healthy child or I'm going to terminate"

is extremely unfair. There are many people out there just waiting
to adopt a child with Down's, and give them a wonderful happy life.
These people KNOW the issues with Downs and are accepting that.

Several women were angry at Olivia for focusing on Down
syndrome as if it represented all disabilities, thereby making IPs'
decisions look frivolous: "This is a huge oversimplification of an
incredibly complicated decision and your tone is demeaning to
anyone who has ever raised a child with life threatening disabilities." Others insisted that she was unfair to IPs who already had to
give up so much control over "their pregnancy": "A surro should
allow the IP to be as 'pregnant' as possible. It is not my choice, my
chance, my child, or my business. Your right to make parenting
decisions is not diminished b/c someone else is carrying your child."
Nevertheless, fully agreeing that surrogacy does not diminish the
IPs' parenthood fails to address the body-self duality, as this reply
to Christina's initial post shows:

> No one is saying you are any less of a parent. But when you involve
> a third party to carry your child, you have to factor in her decisions.
> It is HER body. Surrogates are not emotionless, walking uteruses
> (uteri?) and we have feelings. When a child is in MY body, I will not
> terminate that child unless it is going to die shortly after birth, or
> unless I am going to die unless I terminate.

Again, the solution women can collectively agree on is "finding the
right match" and spelling out everything clearly in the contract.
"You absolutely must be on the same page as your IPs regarding
things like termination and reduction. You can't just sign a contract
and think something won't happen to you."

> I can completely understand if the IPs want to have that option avail-
> able to them. I completely respect that. As a GS, I do not view the IPs
> as "less than." It is their child. BUT as a GS, if I don't believe in abor-
> tion, then how can I go along with it if I clearly play a part? There are
> IPs who also do not believe in terminating at all for any reason and
> want to find a GS who wouldn't terminate either. When a GS doesn't
> want to abort, it isn't that we are trying to take the decision out of
> your hands. We just know it is something we could never be a part of.

As a result of discussions and stories, surrogates collectively conclude: "WE HAVE GOT TO BE MORE SPECIFIC IN WHAT WE
ARE AND ARE NOT WILLING TO DO." This stance offers the
only answer to the body-self problem, which proves to be a much

more challenging division than the separation of gestation and parenthood.

While the learning curve usually results in more carefully worded contracts, it does not preclude the repeated willingness to compromise in order to "make dreams come true." The dreams surrogates refer to are not just the couples' dream for a baby but also the surrogates' for the "perfect couple" and the "perfect journey," or at least for a journey that has greater meaning and transcends utilitarian market considerations.

Honoring the contract

SMO-ers' growing insistence on matching only with like-minded IPs makes even more sense when we understand how unwavering surrogates are about following the contract once it is signed. "If surros say they will terminate or reduce they MUST uphold their end. The IPs would have chosen someone else to carry for them. It is just very, very unfair and wrong," insisted Emmy, who was against terminating a pregnancy unless her life was in danger. "I didn't think it was right to ask for anything outside of the contract," wrote Hannah, who was on bed rest for eleven weeks while carrying twins; she also had a long recovery, and her lost wages were not covered by the contract. There are several reasons for honoring the contract. One is quite pragmatic. "There are plenty of times when one or the other side forgets or misses something in the contract . . . just like I wouldn't want IPs changing things mid-stream, surros shouldn't either."

But there is more to it than the notion that both parties should follow the agreement. "You shouldn't ask for [extras]. I was raised with morals and ethics too and I think when you agree to something you should stick with it." The most common argument for this position integrates the morality of keeping one's word with the morality of rational and well-informed preparation. "I don't think it's too much to ask that a surrogate read through her contract carefully and add what she thinks she might need before she gets pg [pregnant]."

> Everyone should honor what they agreed to in writing, no matter what. . . . Contracts are written for a reason and that is to protect every party in the arrangement and to have a guide for when sensitive issues arise. We all know that when something emotional pops up during your journey, it is hard to see past that emotion and to have effective communication. I am the type of person that always does what I say, whether in writing or verbal, if you don't have your word than what are you worth?

Carefully negotiating the contract and upholding the contractual agreement are ways to assert rationality, reliability, integrity, and also equality with the couple.

Women take collective pride in being not only giving and sensitive but also intelligent and knowledgeable: "If a surro is taken advantage of in the US it's her own fault. There are plenty of ways to educate yourself about what you are getting into and if you as a surro jump into a situation because you are desperate then it's your own fault." SMO members are not sympathetic to uninformed surrogates and condemn what they see as unreliable and erratic behavior. They think of Mary Beth Whitehead and Lashell Baker as women who give surrogates a "bad name."[32]

But while the previous examples showed surrogates' commitment to fairness and mutuality, the following post points to a morality that goes beyond reciprocity. You should never ask for extras, Tanya insisted. "You're supposed to be a good surrogate no matter what the couple does." This morality transcends contractual obligations because one party's behavior is not contingent on the other party's actions. This stance evokes the kind of altruism that characterizes close and loving personal relationships.[33]

Angela was upset that so many IPs went back on their promises and were not willing to make "sacrifices for a relationship." Yet, she wrote, "they could treat me like dog SH*T and they would still get their child and I would still live up to my word. I would take the best care of their baby . . . and LOVE that baby." Ella was treated very badly; she, too, held up her side of the contract. "I know I can hold my head high knowing that I did what I said I would do, and they simply can't. And I am proud of myself for that."

To be sure, there is an element of self-dramatization in posts like these. Selflessness and the commitment to "nurturing life" are the ideal traits of a "great" surrogate. Women compete for the higher moral ground, not only vis-à-vis their couple but in relation to other surrogates. Even though the stories are often about IPs, the real rivals, as well as the real audience, are fellow surrogates. The tacit quest is to be a truly self-sacrificing, giving, and generous woman; other surrogates are sounding board, supporting cast, and fellow contenders. These "performances," to use Goffman's term, although sometimes contentious, bolster women's resolve and help define the ideal morality of surrogacy. Women discursively perform the selves they are "striving to live up to."[34]

These narrative displays of idealized conduct are consistent with Goffman's analysis of stigmatized groups; the perceived stigma of commercial surrogacy puts pressure on surrogates to present idealized generosity.[35] By agreeing that true surrogates do everything they can regardless of how IPs treat them, women collectively turn a possible "stigma symbol," that is, contracting to carry a child for compensation, into a "prestige symbol" of selflessness.[36] They elevate themselves not only above the stigmatized behavior but also above ordinary people and the market logic of exchange. Surrogates also reject the notion that such selflessness is the hallmark of motherhood only. They are sacrificing in order to help others have a family and are often willing to "do whatever it takes" to achieve this goal. Honoring the contract does not preclude the willingness to go above and beyond the agreement; it only bars behavior that would disregard it.

Commitment and sacrifice are also elaborated in discussions about how long one should keep trying to get pregnant for the couple. Surrogates often say they would try more times than they had agreed to in the contract. Not infrequently, women would "keep going" as long as the IPs were willing; they post about their multiyear journeys marked by failed conceptions, miscarriages, and determination. Setting and pursuing goals and not giving up are middle-class values; goal-oriented behavior is considered worthy of respect and reward.[37] "I'm not a quitter," wrote Holly, who was almost more determined than her couple during their twenty-six-month-long journey. Posts about years of trying and going through hardship get sympathetic and admiring responses; fellow surrogates reward perseverance.

These sometimes exaggerated and dramatic posts about generosity and sacrifice are not unlike the self-dramatizations documented by Carol Stack in her study of reciprocal exchange networks in the "Flats."[38] Even though the social context is different, these performances achieve similar ends in both cases: they highlight one's contribution in relation to what one receives. When it comes to personal relationships, being able and willing to give more than one gets is a sign of uncalculating behavior and hence high moral standards.

"it's all about faith, trust, and honor"

Expectations of reciprocity

A bit of dramatization notwithstanding, countless posts testify to the difficulties and risks surrogates encounter and the sacrifices they make. Generosity and sacrifice are commonly understood as the opposite of market logic and are associated with love and altruism, which are essential qualities in building personal ties.[39] Accordingly, no matter how much surrogates insist on fulfilling contractual obligations, they expect their IPs to be supportive, sympathetic, and appreciative, rather than to simply fulfill their contractual promises.

Danielle, who was "extra careful" yet lost a twin pregnancy at fourteen weeks, was upset when her IM reminded her of her contractual obligation to get test results on fetal tissue right after she underwent dilation and curettage (D&C). "I did expect them to be my friend and to be there for me, and not for them to treat me like an employee or a walking incubator."[40] Danielle was hurt by her IM's businesslike reminder of their contractual arrangement when she expected a personal and emotional relationship of support and empathy. A typical response expressed the consensus among surrogates: "a surrogacy contract does not entitle someone to treat you like a human incubator." Surrogates who "care a great deal" about their IPs expect the kind of reciprocity that is inherent in close personal relationships; however, caring behavior cannot be contractually specified or guaranteed.

Like Danielle, surrogates expect their IPs to "be there for them" in diffuse ways. "I just wish my IPs would be more involved or sympathetic," wrote Tina. The couple initially told her they wanted a close friendship, but things changed once she got pregnant, and her e-mails often went unanswered. She did not get much sympathy when she was sick; she did not get any response when she sent ultrasound pictures and recordings of fetal heartbeat. Fellow surrogates advised her not to give up on the relationship; they suggested that the IPs may have been through "too many disappointments" and "guard their hearts." When surrogates look for explanations for IPs' behavior they most frequently point to the psychological impact of infertility.

Charlotte Linde argued that such explanatory systems are popularized forms of originally expert theories that provide "a means for understanding, evaluating, and interpreting experience."[41] If infertility is one of the greatest misfortunes, as surrogates believe, it is bound to have long-lasting psychological implications for those who suffer from it. Accordingly, IPs who had undergone treatments without success or suffered losses must have a hard time learning to trust. Not only do surrogates imagine what it is like to be such a person, they also imagine that by being patient and communicative, and by bearing children for them, they can help

IPs to let their guards down and trust again. This is a powerful fantasy: carrying babies for IPs not only creates families but also restores IPs' psychological health that had been undermined by infertility and failures.

Tina, like most women on SMO, found these explanations compelling and thought of her IPs' behavior as the result of past disappointments. At the urging of fellow surrogates, who tend to believe that discussing feelings is helpful, she told her IPs she wanted to talk about the relationship. They responded by advising her to seek psychological help. At this point the overwhelming agreement on SMO was that Tina should lower her expectations while continuing to do her best, because ultimately surrogacy is not about the surrogate. "If they don't ask you how you are, just e-mail them with the facts." The surrogacy ethic that highlights both independence and selflessness is sometimes expressed in legal language, as in this response to Tina: "there's nothing in your contract that says they have to contact you and become friends with you."

Although surrogates know this, the most painful outcome for them is when IPs cut ties without warning or explanation; such stories may well be overrepresented on SMO precisely because they are so devastating. Jena had a "perfect journey" and received e-mails and pictures for a few months. After not getting any updates for a while Jena eventually contacted her IM's best friend, asking if everything was all right. She was told that "there was no room" for her in her former IM's life. Tessa's intended father went further, saying that "he has no reason to be appreciative." After all, Tessa "did not do anything for them" that she "wasn't paid to do." This was a business transaction; they paid in full and had no reason to be grateful.

When I asked SMO "insiders" about bad stories, I heard variations on this response:

> It happens all the time, unfortunately. IPs tell the surrogates that they will keep in touch, send pictures and give updates. But that is not always the case. Sometimes a journey will go bad and there will be anger . . . and that is why contact is cut off. Other times the IPs just had no intention of updating, they just said they did. It is extremely hurtful. . . . [Surrogates] feel like they were used and tossed aside.[42]

However, surrogates often give IPs the benefit of the doubt. They assume that IPs are busy or guarded but not that they are indifferent not only because SMO-ers are committed to the dream of a "wonderful journey" but also because contractual relationships and friendships share an important element: the parties choose to be obligated. People enter into both contractual and personal relationships as an act of free choice. In contractual relations, they willingly undertake the obligations specified in the contract, but the obligations in personal relationships are diffuse, as Danielle's expectation that her IPs be "there for her" exemplifies.[43] As I argued, surrogates view contract negotiations as the test as well as the basis of a "great match" and often take it for granted that IPs share this view. "Surrogacy is too important and intimate of an experience to walk alongside the wrong people"; surrogates assume that IPs think so, too.

For these women, entering into a surrogacy contract is an expression of how they think of themselves and who they aspire to be: helpful and giving people with high moral standards, a self-selected group of "amazing" women.[44] These self-understandings are enthusiastically elaborated and supported on SMO. This collectively arrived at mindset explains why surrogates do not always have an easy time representing their best interests even though they are well informed. Surrogates' "expressive" approach to contract, to use Hadfield's term, means that they evaluate their options "in light of what the choice would express," that is, their valuation of children, family, and helping others and their desire to be valued, rather than "what future states it would secure" in terms of monetary gain.[45] This expressive view is not in conflict with the learning curve I have described. Surrogates most often want to work out a fair contract, one they consider to be the best foundation for "a wonderful bond" with their IPs, but they do not want to jeopardize that bond and the affective currency it yields by being uncompromising.

Limits of the contract

Most surrogates hope to have a lasting relationship with IPs but as everyone understands, this cannot be achieved by legal means. The limits of the contract are vividly revealed by the following discussion about the utility of contractually regulating the relationship between the surrogate and her IPs after birth. Kendra asked what others thought about including a provision about postbirth contact, given that surrogates would not go to court to enforce it: "Is it just to make us . . . feel better and hopeful that the other party remains true to their word?" The consensus was that it was indeed a "feel good" clause. "They are there to make us all feel secure. But the fact is, it's all about faith, trust and honor."

When IPs keep in touch it confirms that surrogacy creates intimacy, friendship, and lasting emotional bonds. But personal relationships cannot be contractually prescribed, regulated, or enforced. "Putting it in a contract is pointless really. Even if it were legally enforceable, why would you do it? Who wants to be forced to be with someone? If it isn't voluntary then it loses meaning." Samantha expressed the general sentiment: "I would rather have them [keep in touch] on their own free will and love." Without the mutual desire to continue the relationship, "keeping in touch" is not meaningful. "I'm not interested in any fake or contractually (or otherwise) obligated friendship. Of course forming a real and lasting friendship would be ideal but if that does not happen I would not want any party to feel obligated in any way to maintain something that does not exist."

Mina went further and questioned the legitimacy of IPs' postbirth obligation: "I don't feel like I could demand that anyone be obligated to me. I wouldn't ask for it contractually either. If a relationship fell apart then it's over. I might not like it if I were cut off from contact but in the end, I can't imagine forcing the issue." Over time, a more forcefully independent, and somewhat improbable, stance has emerged:

> I EXPECTED nothing. They are NOT my children. No matter how I was treated while pregnant, I expected nothing after the birth. Lucky for me, the parents continued the relationship and I'm tickled to be "Aunt" M. to both boys. I think you set yourself up for failure if you think what you have when you are pregnant will be exactly the same after you deliver. Expect nothing and you will not be disappointed. ;).

Some others were less lucky: "I expected nothing and I am getting what I expected." Surrogates are careful not to sound cynical or bitter, preferring to express confident self-sufficiency: "I didn't go into surrogacy to force a lifelong friendship. . . . I wanted to help an IM have a child. . . . I am thankful for these experiences." Surrogates almost never attempt to enforce postbirth contact even when it was contractually stipulated: "To sue because you aren't given contact. . . . That's stalking and neurotic." They very rarely try to enforce other contractual obligations, including financial ones, even in states where this would be possible. One reason is the legal cost and time investment lawsuits entail. But equally importantly, surrogates want to regain their peace of mind, assured that they did "a wonderful thing" for their IPs; they do not want to prolong the pain and bitterness.

> My opinion, suing is worthless . . . unless you have limitless money
> to afford the time, cost and energy of a lawsuit . . . there isn't much
> that can be done in regards to the contract. Ironic since everyone
> says how important contracts are. But it takes hours of legal work,
> depositions, travel and so on to pursue a case, especially if you decide
> to throw emotional distress into the mix. Personally, i think therapy,
> writing your story and being heard are the best recourse in situations
> where IPs screw you. In the end you have to figure out how to make
> peace with it all.

Surrogates most often have no alternative to seeking peace and closure when things go wrong. As I documented in Chapter 2, women
struggle to refocus on the shared aim: "letting go of the negative
feelings and seeing the positives—you helped bring a child into the
world."

The ultimate limitation of the contract, however, lies in the fact
that no surrogate would force responsibility for the baby on unwilling IPs. "I found out on Monday that I am carrying twins. I also
found out that my IM doesn't feel that she can care for twins. . . .
This is devastating," wrote Amelia, who was carrying for a single
woman. Surrogates are baffled at such a development; they assume
that people who were unable to have children are delighted to have
their dream come true. "What is with all the IMs lately?? This is
the 3rd one I have heard of in a week that is just going to walk away
from their child(ren)." Many others expressed hope that after she
recovers from the shock of having twins Amelia's IM will want the
babies. This did not happen. In the ensuing prolonged discussions,
however, no one suggested that Amelia should in any way force
her IM to take responsibility for the babies. Amelia found new IPs
for the twins while still pregnant, and everyone agreed this was a
"wonderful outcome."

Some other IPs walked away because they split up, had marital problems, did not want triplets, or realized a bit too late how
expensive surrogacy was. As far as it is possible to know from these
discussions, at least some of these IPs had used donor gametes. But
no matter when and why IPs refuse to take the baby, SMO-ers never
make the argument that IPs should be required to fulfill their contractual obligation and take the baby they do not want. IPs insist
that "legal protection for their parentage" be included in the contract; there is no equivalent insistence by surrogates about legal
protection *from* responsibility for the baby.[46]

Contracts often specify who will take care of the babies if both
IPs die before the birth but do not address the what-if scenario of IPs

changing their mind. Surrogates assume that IPs are desperate to have a baby; they also assume responsibility when IPs do not. Surrogates found adoptive parents for babies the IPs rejected, including ones with Down syndrome. In one famous case, an older couple failed to claim the triplets (conceived with donor gametes) their surrogate gave birth to until two weeks after the birth. They also lied to Sally, the surrogate, about their marital status. Sally took the babies home after the couple failed to show up and decided that her IPs were not good parent material. She went to court and gained custody and subsequently found adoptive parents for the babies; the whole process took about six months, during which time she cared for the triplets.

Surrogates want to create families by carrying babies for deserving people who will love and care for them. IPs should desperately want the baby; the surrogate dream cannot accommodate the reality of people changing their minds or being irresponsible about the "precious life" surrogates help create. The contract is ultimately useless when IPs are no longer eager to have the baby.

In their best-selling book, *Habits of the Heart,* Bellah and his collaborators theorized that the troubling social problem in the contemporary United States "is that too much of the purely contractual structure of the economic and bureaucratic world is becoming an ideological model for personal life. . . . The prevalence of contractual intimacy and procedural cooperation . . . is what threatens to obscure the ideals of both personal virtue and public good."[47] What we witness on SMO, however, is a less simple and one-directional phenomenon. Contractual structures are imposed on baby making; yet we see women striving to turn procedural cooperation into reciprocal care. Reading SMO threads reveals the creative negotiation, expression, and perpetuation of "virtue" through contractual intimacy.

Surrogates' contractual choices may not be a "choice about the future," or at least not in terms of future gain, but "a way of expressing something in the present."[48] Through the contract, surrogates express themselves as caring women; they also express their commitment to providing "deserving" people with a much-wanted child. Conventional legal theory with its utility- and profit-maximizing rationality does not account for these choices and does not take into consideration other forms of value and other ways of accounting.

Surrogates' discussions about contract negotiations shed light on how emotions and imagination inform choices and illuminate the fact that contracts cannot regulate emotional valuation. I am not making the argument that rationality and emotionality, or contract and friendship, are antagonistic; rather, I consider all these often incommensurable considerations part of the intricate decision-making process that produces contracts and relationships.

Surrogates would agree with Richard Epstein's claim that in surrogacy voluntary exchange "promotes human welfare," even if some exchange is offensive to some people.[49] They would, however, disagree with his claim that enforceable contracts are sufficient to guarantee "good outcomes" between rational actors.[50] Epstein's assumption that "the terms and conditions of the relationship can be fully explained . . . to the potential surrogate" is problematic when we consider the empirical evidence. Clearly, the contractual relationship is by no means the only relationship surrogates care about, and while the terms of the contract are generally clear to surrogates, the terms of personal relationship with IPs cannot be fully predicted or explained.[51] Epstein's assertion that greater gain justifies giving up some freedom and enduring some restrictions is also empirically problematic.[52] Surrogates frequently endure restrictions and even hardship before they see any "gain," and there is ample evidence that they do not define, nor try to calculate, gain the way Epstein assumes.

Contracts are clearly not a simple matter of conveying information or allocating mutually calculable benefits. As I documented, SMO-ers have access to information and advocate an ethic of responsibility, which includes researching surrogacy before matching. Legal scholars' ideas of mutual benefits are not what surrogates call a "win-win." Benefits in the legal sense are based on costs versus gains calculation, impossible to compute in surrogacy, even if surrogates were interested in such computations.

First, it often takes many months to achieve pregnancy, during which time surrogates get reimbursed for expenses but do not receive any compensation; compensation typically starts at either the first positive pregnancy blood test or the first fetal heartbeat. Yet, gestational surrogates take hormones for weeks and often undergo repeated transfer cycles, traditional surrogates undergo artificial insemination, and both spend time attending various medical appointments before they receive any compensation.

Second, potential complications make surrogates' pregnancy-related costs impossible to predict. As much as women increasingly learn to protect themselves better by not allowing their lost wages to be capped, they cannot fully shield themselves from adverse consequences. For example, employed surrogates may be laid off if they miss too many days of work because of the pregnancy. In fact, some women lost their jobs and had to face long-term financial and emotional consequences. Nor are the costs of health risks calculable; many surrogates developed diabetes and high blood pressure or had other long-term health issues due to the many rounds of hormone treatments or complications at birth.[53]

Third, costs and benefits are not only monetary but also physical and emotional, and thus incommensurable. Countless threads conclude that having higher compensation is not worth it if the IPs are uncaring and do not want contact or cut ties after birth. When IPs fail to pay the compensation, fees, or medical bills it can be financially costly for surrogates, but the emotional "cost" of disappointment is also hard to bear. To surrogates, mutual benefit means a mutually caring and helping relationship, or at least a mutually honest and respectful one.

My findings indicate that contrary to conventional contract theory, surrogates and IPs do not always see the contract the same way and are not always trying to achieve the same goals, and they often do not fully realize this during negotiations. Both parties focus on creating a baby; for IPs, the baby is the goal and the benefit. But for surrogates, the goal is a much more complex matter. Women expect to gain emotional satisfaction from surrogacy as well as affective currency and fair financial compensation from their IPs. If, as my data show, surrogates are more invested in "making people's dream of parenthood come true" than securing personal gain, some of the things that are important to them are not regulated by the contract because they do not belong to the realm of contractual relations. Thus, contrary to Epstein's claim, "the terms and conditions of the relationship" are not a simple matter because they do not coincide with the terms and conditions of the contract.[54]

IPs do not always think they owe affective "payment" to the surrogate. As SMO discussions show, women are satisfied when they are appreciated and devastated when the IPs deny their sacrifice and cut ties.[55] Women are contented when they are "on the same page" with their IPs, not simply as far as the contract is concerned but also about the meaning of surrogacy. But in the end, and because of the support and empathy SMO-ers provide one another, emotional dividends are somewhat separable from IPs' appreciation. Surrogacy affirms the value of children and family, and thus validates surrogates' own life choices and priorities, and valorizes their otherwise taken for granted fertility.[56] Surrogates gain recognition and appreciation from fellow SMO-ers, who console them and cheer them on. SMO membership thus pays emotional dividends; women feel supported and understood and take pride in being strong and giving.

Notes

1. SMO-ers discuss and recommend lawyers, and lawyers gain no favor among surrogates (or on SMO) unless they represent the surrogates' best interests. For example, after a question about an unusually worded contract, a responder pointed out, "I have never heard of this lawyer in 6yrs in this world [i.e., the surrogacy world]!! She must not be one people recommend!"
2. Of the 234 surrogates who voted on an informal poll about all-inclusive fees, forty percent said theirs would be between 30,000 and 40,000 dollars, thirty six percent would have higher fees, and twenty six percent would have lower ones.
3. Extras usually include fees for some or all of the following, but this is not a complete list: invasive procedures, C-section, loss of reproductive organs, multifetal pregnancy, selective reduction, transfer, canceled cycle (when the surrogate took medications and the transfer was canceled for some reason), life insurance policy, maternity clothes allowance, daycare for surrogates' children when she is going to appointments or is incapacitated due to the pregnancy, housekeeper in case surrogate needs it, reimbursement of lost wages in case the surrogate was unable to work for some other pregnancy-related reason.
4. Many IPs prefer all-inclusive fees as long as they do not include all what-ifs. IPs often worry that the extras in the "base fees and extras" could add up and cost too much.
5. Compensation may be paid in four or five chunks: at the confirmation of pregnancy, at the end of each trimester, and after the birth. Fewer installments are considered odd.
6. Viviana A. Zelizer, "How I Became a Relational Economic Sociologist and What Does That Mean?" *Politics & Society* 40, no. 2 (2012): 157.
7. Ibid., 152.
8. Jonathan Parry and Maurice Bloch, eds., *Money and the Morality of Exchange* (New York: Cambridge University Press, 1989), 9.
9. For example, Berkhout argues that the contractual relationship symbolizes the objectification of surrogates, and thus diminishes their self-respect. Suze G. Berkhout, "Buns in the Oven: Objectification, Surrogacy, and Women's Autonomy," *Social Theory and Practice* 34, no. 1 (2008): 96–97. Melinda Roberts asserted that contract surrogacy

equals "the commercial disposal and acquisition of children" and is thus against the best interests of the child. Melinda A. Roberts, "Good Intentions and a Great Divide: Having Babies by Intending Them," *Law and Philosophy* 12, no. 3 (1993): 299.

10. Elizabeth S. Scott, "Surrogacy and the Politics of Commodification," *Law and Contemporary Problems* 72 (2009): 109–46. See also Kimberly Krawiec, "Altruism and Intermediation in the Market for Babies," *Washington and Lee Law Review* 66 (2009): 43.

11. Two early defenders of surrogacy contracts were Lori Andrews, *New Conceptions* (New York: Ballantine, 1985) and Carmel Shalev, *Birth Power: The Case for Surrogacy* (New Haven, CT: Yale University Press, 1989). Also see Richard Epstein, "Surrogacy: The Case for Full Contractual Enforcement," *Virginia Law Review* 81, no. 8 (1995): 2305–41; Christine Kerian, "Surrogacy: A Last Resort Alternative for Infertile Women or a Commodification of Women's Bodies and Children?" *Wisconsin Women's Law Journal* 12, no. 1 (1997): 113–66; Hugh V. McLachlan and Kim Swales, "Commercial Surrogate Motherhood and the Alleged Commodification of Children: A Defense of Legally Enforceable Contracts," *Law and Contemporary Problems* 72 (2009): 91–107; Peter Schuck, "Some Reflections on the Baby M Case," *Georgetown Law Journal* 76, no. 5 (1987): 1793–810.

12. Kerian, "Surrogacy"; Schuck, "Some Reflections"; Richard A. Posner, "The Ethics and Economics of Enforcing Contracts of Surrogate Motherhood," *Journal of Contemporary Health Law and Policy* 5 (1989): 21.

13. Epstein, "Surrogacy," 2312.

14. Ibid., 2318.

15. Melvin Aron Eisenberg, "The Limits of Cognition and the Limits of Contract," *Stanford Law Review* 47, no. 2 (1995): 212.

16. Ibid., 211–12.

17. Ibid.

18. Gillian Hadfield, "An Expressive Theory of Contract: From Feminist Dilemmas to a Reconceptualization of Rational Choice in Contract Law," *University of Pennsylvania Law Review* 146, no. 5 (1998): 1259–60.

19. Ibid., 1261.

20. Ibid., 1262.

21. Anne C. Dailey, "Imagination and Choice," *Law and Social Inquiry* 35, no. 1 (2010): 175–216.

22. Gerald L. Clore, "For Love or Money: Some Emotional Foundations of Rationality," *Chicago-Kent Law Review* 80, no. 3 (2005): 1151–65; Dailey, "Imagination and Choice"; Viviana A. Zelizer, *The Purchase of Intimacy* (Princeton, NJ: Princeton University Press, 2005).

23. Despite widespread beliefs that surrogates may change their mind about relinquishing the baby, surrogates themselves take it for granted that sane surrogates never do this, unless some serious problems occur (e.g., IPs do not show up at the birth, IPs do not want the baby, or some other indication that they are irresponsible). There have been a few

such cases; nonpayment is never considered a reason for not handing the baby over to IPs.

24. John Boli, "The Economic Absorption of the Sacred," in *Rethinking Materialism: Perspectives on the Spiritual Dimension of Economic Behavior*, ed. Robert Wuthnow (Grand Rapids, MI: Eerdmans), 93–115; Robert Wuthnow, *Meaning and Moral Order* (Berkeley: University of California Press, 1987).

25. Patricia Ewick and Susan S. Silbey, "Conformity, Contestation, and Resistance: An Account of Legal Consciousness," *New England Law Review* 26 (1992): 741.

26. Joanna, e-mail communication, 4 May 2010.

27. Ava, e-mail communication, 10 April 2010. I found that surrogates very often use love metaphors to describe their expectations as well as their relationship with and feelings toward their IPs. Elly Teman documented similar emotions among Israeli surrogates in *Birthing a Mother: The Surrogate Body and the Pregnant Self* (Berkeley: University of California Press, 2010).

28. In countless threads surrogates exchange stories about comments they get that they "do it for the money." Repeat surrogates often advise one another not to mind: "After the first time, everyone will assume you are doing it for the money. I guess we get one time for them to think we are just trying to help and after that, we're all about the money. I have tried everything I can think of: witty remarks, sarcastic remarks, remarks meant to educate. . . . People will not change their minds about what we are doing."

29. PTO is a policy that provides a bank of hours in which the employer pools sick days, vacation days, and personal days that employees are allowed to use as the need or desire arises. Unlike more traditional leave plans, PTO plans are more flexible because they do not distinguish employee absences from personal days, vacation days, or sick days. Upon employment, the company determines how many PTO hours will be allotted per year and a "rollover" policy. Some companies let PTO hours accumulate for only a year, and unused hours disappear at year-end.

30. Pre-embryos (surrogates call them embryos or embies) are frozen in "straws," and once thawed they cannot be refrozen. In this post the surrogate is conflicted because unless all three are transferred one is "wasted."

31. Teman, *Birthing a Mother*, 55–56.

32. Whitehead was the traditional surrogate who changed her mind in the famous Baby M custody case in 1986. Lashell Baker, a two-time surrogate and mother of four, carried twins for the Kehoes (both egg and sperm were "donated"), a couple she met on SMO in 2009. At the guardianship hearing Baker learned that Amy Kehoe was on medication for paranoid disorder and also had a past drug conviction—facts that Amy Kehoe had kept from Baker. Baker withdrew her consent

and was awarded custody because Michigan law is opposed to commercial surrogacy and the Kehoes were genetically unrelated to the twins. Lashell tried to explain on SMO that she never planned to keep the babies, but after discovering these facts about Amy she felt this was the responsible thing to do: "So, if I am a bad surrogate because I choose the safety of my surrobabies over my name, then I am a bad surrogate. . . . I think that they deceived me because they knew that any other surrogate including myself would not work with them knowing the present mental state and criminal state of the couple." Although surrogates normally agree that honesty is essential, "keeping the baby" is such a taboo that the great majority of the women who posted on the very long thread (it contained 369 posts when the moderator closed it) condemned Lashell. Some of them used very strong language, calling her "worse than a hoe." Amy Kehoe started her own threads and received many sympathetic and supportive responses; women also collected money for her to help with legal fees. However, the Kehoes did not pursue the case, posting that it was a lost cause.

33. Howard Bahr and Kathleen S. Bahr, "Families and Self-Sacrifice: Alternative Models and Meanings for Family Theory," *Social Forces* 79, no. 4 (2001): 1231–58.
34. Erving Goffman, *The Presentation of Self in Everyday Life* (New York: Doubleday, 1959), 19.
35. Erving Goffman, *Stigma: Notes on the Management of Spoiled Identity* (New York: Simon and Schuster, 1963).
36. Ibid., 43.
37. Linda L. Layne, *Motherhood Lost. A Feminist Account of Pregnancy Loss in America* (New York: Routledge, 2003).
38. Carol B. Stack, *All Our Kin: Strategies for Survival in a Black Community* (New York: Basic Books, 1975), 38–39.
39. Kenneth Boulding, *The Economy of Love and Fear* (Belmont, CA: Wadsworth, 1973); Bellah et al., *Habits of the Heart: Individualism and Commitment in American Life* (Berkeley: University of California Press, 1985).
40. Surrogates often say they are just the incubator, the oven, or the babysitter but do not take it kindly when people treat them as such.
41. Charlotte Linde, "Explanatory Systems in Oral Life Stories," in *Cultural Models in Language and Thought*, ed. Dorothy Holland and Naomi Quinn (Cambridge: University of Cambridge Press, 1987), 351–52.
42. Joanna, e-mail communication, 4 May 2010.
43. David M. Schneider, *American Kinship: A Cultural Account* (Englewood Cliffs, NJ: Prentice-Hall, 1968), 61.
44. They often call each other "amazing" and "selfless" even though they may disclaim being special themselves. Surrogates sometimes report being surprised when praised by outsiders. However, by asserting that carrying babies and taking risks for others is not hard for *them*, they in fact elevate themselves above the majority for whom it would be.
45. Hadfield, "Expressive Theory of Contract," 1237.

46. Israeli state regulation protects surrogates; IPs have a legal obligation to assume responsibility for the baby.

47. Bellah et al., *Habits of the Heart*, 126.

48. Hadfield, "Expressive Theory of Contract," 1265.

49. Epstein, "Surrogacy," 2312.

50. Ibid., 2318.

51. Ibid.

52. Ibid., 2335.

53. Due to multiple pre-embryo transfers, surrogates quite often carry twins and sometimes triplets, and such pregnancies and deliveries entail more risks. Many surrogates had Cesarean deliveries and prolonged recovery time. Repeat gestational surrogates undergo many rounds of hormone treatments during their journeys; transfers fail, and each cycle involves a protocol of hormones, the long-term side effects of which are not known.

54. Epstein, "Surrogacy," 2318.

55. Teman, in *Birthing a Mother*, found the same to be true for Israeli surrogates who initially undertake surrogacy for monetary gain. Yet during the pregnancy they increasingly adopt the gift rhetoric and worry about the future of their relationship with their IMs. Monetary payment, guaranteed by state regulation, did nothing to alleviate their sense of disappointment when the relationship with the IPs soured.

56. My argument is not that surrogates carry babies for others in order to validate their own life choices, rather that surrogacy affirms the values and practices they hold dear.

Chapter 4

MONEY

This chapter documents the ways in which surrogates see and understand the role and significance of money in surrogacy arrangements. First, I explore discussions about motivations, compensation, and also definitions of altruism and its coexistence with monetary rewards. Second, I show the ways in which surrogates think about the connections between money, fairness, and appreciation. Third, I document surrogates' discussions of cost-saving ideas and practices and their debates about the price of experience and the savings it represents. Fourth, I discuss the ways in which surrogates' claims about the uniqueness of the relationship with their couple are negotiated through financial practices.

"it's not about money"

Money and motivation

Surrogates are in agreement that women who go through hardship to make the intended parents' dream of parenthood come true deserve compensation. Money, however, is not what defines surrogacy for surrogates.

> So many [people] who do such an amazing thing in helping others and they get paid and nobody bats an eye and yet when it's . . . surrogacy, everyone thinks we make a fortune, or they look at us like we are money hungry . . . Of course for most of us if not all this is absolutely not the case.

Intended mothers sometimes assure SMO-ers that surrogates, just like babies, are priceless: "Let me first say I feel comp is more than justified and if you asked me what a fair amount would be for the child who now owns my heart, I swear there is not a number high enough." Countless discussions elaborate that compensation is well deserved but is not the main motivation for becoming a surrogate:

> My "reward" for doing it for a stranger is the money and also know-ing I helped create a family. Nothing I could ever do could give me the feeling of joy like hearing my IM's voice when I tell her "it worked we are pregnant", seeing my IPs face at the birth of their child and children, seeing my surro baby and knowing "I" carried him and her for their family. The feeling is INDESCRIBABLE. I've NEVER done something so GRATIFYING, so WONDERFUL, so AMAZING, so UNBELIEVABLE. How can you put a price on what we do? You can't. The comp is to "help" our family, just like we "helped" another family. We not only put our life on "hold" for over a year, stick needles in our body for 4 months. . . . Not to mention risking our life and putting our family through a lot. . . . All of this for in most cases a stranger. And people get all bent out of shape about us being compensated!! . . . And "baby selling" will not work, because you can't sell what is not yours.

> As a 3x compensated SM, I do feel that SMs deserve to be compen-sated. I also believe that no amount of compensation is enough. There is no amount of money that can repay someone for bringing a child into this world. Unfortunately, I think some (not all) IPs think that they are simply paying for a service. I think that if most SMs felt the same way, their fees would be much higher. The only thing that can truly compensate me for being a surrogate mother is genuine gratitude, which does not cost a red dime.

Responses echo these views: "yeah I get something back . . . a little more than money . . . I got to know a great family, whom I have become attached to, I have gotten a great feeling of pride . . . maybe that is all the PAYMENT I need." Surrogates get irritated by the fairly constant focus on money but often remind one another that the appropriate response is pity; people who focus on money do not understand love and giving. "People just can't comprehend this type of unselfish love, concern, and giving exists. So the EASY answer is 'it's the money'. Sometimes I get a little angry with people who just don't get it. . . . Then I feel sorry for them."

After reading an article about how surrogates need the money for their livelihood, Tiffany vented on the boards: "This makes me

crazy! Most people I have informed about my being a GS have commented on doing it to 'pay the bills'! Even my own mother! I truly
believe that there is soooooo much ignorance out there!" Dianne
was not spared either: "My sister-in-law told me to go 'sell more
babies.' . . . When I told my mom I was pregnant with my second
surrogacy she said, 'Dianne, do you like money THAT much?' I just
turned and walked away. Sometimes that's all you can do."

In a fairly typical post Jennifer emphatically rejected the notion
that just because she received compensation, she engaged in a purely
economic transaction: "In my surrogacies, the relationships always
emphasized love, respect, trust and appreciation for my family and
ours in return to my IPs." Love and trust indicate strong positive
affect that typically characterizes intimate relationships. Surrogates
are emphatic about marking relationship boundaries by listing love,
trust, and gratitude among the rewards they receive. Mutual appreciation and respect are the affective currencies Jennifer and many
other surrogates evoke in order to differentiate their transactions
with IPs from market exchange.

In the previous chapters I argued that surrogates think of surrogacy as a personal relationship, albeit one that is based on careful contract negotiations. Because contract negotiations are by
definition businesslike but personal relationships are not, women
are careful to mark the difference between these two types of relationship and, hence, two competing moral definitions of surrogacy.
They do this mainly through monetary distinctions; forms and definitions of payments are carefully matched with the social ties surrogates have or hope to have with their couple.[1] "To the extent that
two relations are easily confused, weighty in their consequences for
participants and/or significantly different in their implications for
third parties, participants . . . devote exceptional effort to marking
what the relationship is and is not."[2]

The relations with which surrogacy is very often confused are
bodily commodification, on the one hand, and motherhood, on the
other. Surrogates make sustained efforts to distinguish between the
different possible interpretations of the relationships of surrogacy
and mark their boundaries. Zelizer argued that "people manage the
mingling of economic activity and intimacy by creating, enforcing, and renegotiating extensive differentiation among social ties,
their boundaries, and their appropriate matching with commercial
media."[3] Making these distinctions is highly important to surrogates and typically requires quite a bit of creative effort.

Surrogates thus engage in "relational work" through carefully matching transactions with their definition of the relationship with intended parents. Chapter 3 documented the distinctions surrogates make between *reimbursements* for expenses, *fees* for various contingencies that offer protection from adverse financial consequences, and *compensation* for pain and suffering. None of these monies are understood as price. Surrogates mark the difference between their practices and sexual services and bodily commodification in general by insisting that the payment is not for gestational services but compensation for pain, time, and effort. They also contrast price with pricelessness: "Prostitution isn't priceless . . . having a child is! Any women can be a prostitute . . . but it takes a good person who cares about others to be a surrogate."

SMO-ers frequently take up the issue of the implied moral stigma: "It's difficult as a surrogate because you are often treated poorly without anyone doing their homework. It gets old really fast when you are treated like you are doing something immoral." Feminist critics have also called surrogacy "reproductive prostitution."[4] Prostitution is a very evocative term.[5] It refers not only to immoral or unethical conduct but also, as Simmel put it, to "purchasable satisfaction which rejects any relationship."[6] The prostitution metaphor is thus doubly insulting to surrogates: it questions both their morality and their uniqueness and negates the personal nature of their relationship with the intended parents.

Surrogates reject accusations of commodification, whether of babies, women, or gestation. These distinctions matter because the consequences are weighty indeed, although not symmetrically so for surrogates and IPs. IPs may frame surrogacy as paid service without negative moral implications, although they are just as appalled by perceptions of baby buying as surrogates are by accusations of baby selling. Surrogates, however, rarely if ever embrace the service model; being a service provider still situates surrogacy in the world of work.[7]

Surrogates often have an impressively subtle reading of not simply money practices but other everyday meanings that reflect the divide between personal relations and employment, between weekends of private life and weekdays of work. "IM would typically only call me and email during the week during her work hours. . . . this is why I began to feel like maybe she thought of me as an employee and not a friend," explained Molly. Annabelle also paid attention to timing: "The one thing I didn't like is being told to call every Friday to check in. . . . I felt like an employee having to give a weekly report." Barbara understood her IMs' unwilling- ness to spend time with her on weekends as an indication that they were not friends. "IM seemed always to be out of town visiting relatives . . . [on weekends when she] was in town, she was always doing stuff with her friends . . . and she would always tell me about [it] on Monday morning. How nice." When surrogates feel excluded from the private life of their IPs, they take it as a sign that they are not valued as an equal partner in the journey.

Valuation is an especially sensitive issue because surrogates are compensated. Even though money changes hands in many trans- actions that are not sales, payment is a form of valuation associ- ated with markets and commodification. References to feeling like an employee always have negative connotations on SMO because employee is an essentially unequal social identity in relation to the employer and in the social structure in general.[8] Because equality is an important concern for surrogates in compensated journeys, much of valuation—appreciation, thankfulness, consideration, care—is channeled, contested, and affirmed through financial negotiations and arrangements, highlighting the role of money in surrogacy arrangements.

Media representations of surrogacy highlight money, too. In the movie *Spanglish* (Columbia Pictures, 2004), the attractive house- keeper is told, "You could make a fortune at *surrogate* pregnancy." News stories are often titled "Wombs for Rent" or "Babies for Sale."[9] At the conservative end of the journalistic spectrum, Charlotte Allen concluded her otherwise well-researched article, "Womb for Rent," with the following rhetorical question: "You have to wonder whether the difference between Theresa Ericson's Ukraine-based baby-selling ring and ordinary US-based surrogacy, in which the baby is ordered up in advance for the same amount of money, isn't one of degree rather than kind."[10]

Over the years, negative views of US surrogacy have been muted and even overshadowed by the growing negative media coverage of Indian surrogacy. Indian surrogates are always depicted as poor and desperate for money, while US surrogates are increasingly portrayed as altruistic.[11] Still, in public representations and private remarks money is often singled out as the defining feature of surrogacy, even if surrogates are not portrayed as destitute. Surrogates encounter comments about money from acquaintances, neighbors, their chil- dren's teachers, even family members and friends, as I discussed in Chapter 2.

SMO-ers often report that total strangers have no inhibition asking them how much money they get. It is against this backdrop of fairly constant questions and comments about money that surrogates emphasize nonmarket considerations such as empathy for their couple and creating a much wished-for life. "I think people squirm when they think about money changing hands in conjunction with human life being created. . . . we are giving them the chance to have a child they couldn't have." It is not so much that they are "downplaying" monetary considerations, as Ragoné argued; rather, they are responding to relentless and often one-sided assumptions about their financial motivations.[12]

The meaning of surrogacy is also at stake. Lay people and social critics may express it differently, but the emphasis on money frames surrogacy as a commodity exchange.[13] Even when surrogates' morality is not called into question directly, their motivation is.

Although SMO-ers dislike comments about money, they repeatedly bring up money matters in their own discussions. My findings indicate that they do so for interrelated reasons: SMO discussions enable surrogates to collectively respond to criticism without denying the importance of money and allow them to make sense of their complex motivations and to situate money in the relational rather than in the business context of surrogacy.

Discussions from the early 2000s and posts reminiscing about first journeys indicate that some women did not know about compensation when they first looked into surrogacy. Surrogates dwell on these memories because they provide irrefutable proof that they are not "in it for the money": "When I first investigated being a surrogate, I went and spoke to a local atty who specializes in surrogacy. She explained the legalities, the meds and the compensation. When she started talking about the compensation, I almost fell out of my chair. . . . I had no clue that people earned money to be a surrogate."

Many others write about being similarly surprised: "I remember when I started researching surrogacy and thought, 'Wow, we can get paid, too.'"[14] Since those early days money has become a much better known feature of surrogacy. Although surrogates hate it when outsiders assume they are motivated by money, they periodically start polls about motivation, sometimes directly asking, "Did you get into surrogacy for money?" Many women who voted on these polls also posted more detailed answers; most expressed unease with having to choose a main reason. "Why does it only have to be one motivation or the other?"

Another poll on compensation asked "Was your surrogacy mainly about money?" and responses similarly expressed dissatisfaction with the question: "I marked yes, only because I would NOT do this for no comp. Some people may see that as 'doing it for the money' some may not. It's not the only reason, but it is definitely a deciding factor." Others elaborated more:

> So . . . it's hard to put a yes or no answer. Would i do a free surrogacy? Yes, for family or like family. So money would NOT be the reason to do surrogacy. For strangers . . . yes i would ask a fee. . . . Do i do surrogacy JUST for the money? NO. . . . In my heart i know i do surrogacy for the love of it. To help make a family and in return the gift i get is in my heart and know the money is a bonus. . . . I think most surros just ask for a figure they are comfortable with and that they know most IPs can afford. And most are willing to lower that for the right IPs.

Surrogates repeatedly articulate that the reasons are complex and that being paid does not mean they are "doing it for the money": "For most of us money is a factor, just not the main one." Responses indicate money is part of an intricate calculation that combines altruism, reciprocity, emotional benefits, and rewards for the surrogate's family:

> My motivation is simply to help a couple achieve their dream of having their own child. . . . I don't want to be pregnant for the attention or for the financial gain. I just want to help a loving couple. . . . I am not saying that the financial aspect doesn't play a role, it does, but . . . it is not a motivation.

> I honestly couldn't say I would do it for nothing. . . . surrogacy . . . is hard! Hard on the surro, hard on her family and hard on her finances if she has a difficult pregnancy. So I did have to consider the $$ motivation. . . . I can't wait to be a part of this wonderful world called surrogacy. . . . I can't wait to be able to take my children to Disney world as a gift for their patience during the surrogacy. I wouldn't have been able to say the last statement without the comp being part of the equation.

> the way my IM looks at it, we are helping each other. They get to have the baby they dream of, I get to take my family on a trip to Disney world, . . . I guess I could have walked away when I realized that they didn't have enough money saved up, but what is worth more to me? A little extra money, or that lifetime friendship/feeling that I will get?

Others explain that they "did it for the money" the first time, although they are quick to add that the money was for a special project, not for livelihood. Women also point out that even though money was their primary motivation, they were still helping couples become family. The following is a fairly typical expression of this stance:

> I admit that I did it for the money the first time. . . . Not that we necessarily needed the extra money, but I wanted to pay my student loans off altogether. . . . This second go around, I am investing it into my SO's business venture. . . . I look at it as an investment in my family and what is wrong with that? I'm darn good at carrying babies and why can't I get paid to help those that can't?

Becoming a surrogate in order to make ends meet is very much condemned; SMO-ers contend that such desperate women cannot possibly be good surrogates. They all agree that good surrogates are informed and responsible; destitute women do not have the means to become well informed, neither can they afford to take care of themselves the way surrogates should. Beyond this, however, surrogates increasingly do not see monetary motivation as a real problem if the surrogate behaves responsibly.

Shifting priorities

In fact, many women confessed that money was an incentive for them. Almost all surrogates who said that money was the initial motivation described the subsequent change in their priorities much like Becky: "I did it the first time for the money. Obviously I got a WHOLE lot more out of it than money. . . . I did it for the $$ and helping was a total bonus . . . only it got turned around for me . . . helping was amazing and the money was a total bonus!" Leah similarly underlined the shift in priorities as her interest in surrogacy progressed to commitment:

> Yes, money was a part of the initial decision to look into surrogacy. BUT the reasons to follow through with it and put your heart, soul, and body into something so spectacular FAR outweigh the importance on money. The money does help soften the blow to the time our family will be apart, when mommy will be crazy sick with morning sickness, the cold shoulder DH will get when I am "off limits" before, during, and after, etc. etc. . . . and after all is said and done . . . I think I'll feel just as lucky to have been a part of this as my IPs are to have their dreams come true.

Teman documented comparable shifts among Israeli surrogates, all of them single mothers and most of them quite poor, who had become surrogates in order to earn extra money. Yet even though money was their primary reason for surrogacy, and unlike in the United States, being paid for carrying a baby is not stigmatized in Israel, all the surrogates commented on how money had become much less important over time. The desire to achieve pregnancy and deliver a healthy baby had taken precedence over remuneration, and the feeling of accomplishment was tied to providing the couple with a baby, not to making extra money. This is an especially interesting comparison because critics of surrogacy in the United States often assert that surrogates' claims about shifting priorities are nothing more than a socially acceptable way to explain their actions and mask their real, that is, pecuniary, motivations.

Given that payment to surrogates is not considered problematic or stigmatized in Israel, there is no reason for Israeli surrogates to deny their financial motivation or talk about shifting priorities, unless their thinking about the meaning of surrogacy had actually changed over time. Sharmila Rudrappa argued that although Indian garment workers in Bangalore became surrogates for the monetary reward, they found moral meanings in giving life. "Surrogacy was also more meaningful for the women than other forms of paid employment. Because babies are life-affirming in ways garments are obviously not, surrogacy allowed women to assert their moral worth."[15]

There is empirical evidence that moral reevaluations and shifting priorities are real in the United States as well. Rene Almeling found that egg donors who were interested in monetary compensation also often came to see donation as helping others or felt somewhat ambivalent about their focus on remuneration.[16] Jennifer Haylett documented that egg donors who were initially motivated by financial compensation often came to adopt a relational perspective when they were picked by potential recipients.[17]

After being matched with an anonymous couple, and with help from the fertility clinic, egg donors engaged in a one-sided relational process whereby their priorities shifted from remuneration to helping a couple become parents. These prospective egg donors equated the amounts of money potential recipient couples spent on the process with good parenting. Surrogates similarly see the amount of money spent on attempts at pregnancy as an indication that IPs are deserving.[18] The more IPs pay for assisted reproductive technologies, including what they had spent on fertility specialists and IVF before matching with the surrogate, the more SMO-ers see them as worthy, committed parents who deserve a child.

Ironically, the more surrogates learn about what it takes to go through the process, and the more realistic they become about risks, the more monetary motivations take a backseat. "The first time I considered [money], yes. When I actually moved forward and took action to be a surrogate, no. By the time I knew more about it, I understood the financial risk it would pose to my family. No amount of comp is worth gambling that," Marcia concluded. The more she learned about the physical and financial risks, the more she realized that money could not be the main reason for her to become a surrogate; the compensation alone would not be worth taking these risks. By the time she made a commitment to her couple, money, although important, was not her primary incentive. Gaby similarly found that money had become less important as actual hardships multiplied, even as she acknowledged the importance of money:

> after a termination, a miscarriage, one failed cycle, two cancelled and now being 14.5 weeks PG [pregnant], it's not about the money so much anymore. . . . I want their and my "happy ending;" a baby in their arms and a brother or sister for their son and for me, to be able to live with the life-long gift, that I help bring a baby in to the world for such wonderful people BUT the money is a great help and I won't ever say [that] I'd do it for free!

Thus, difficult journeys with repeated failures and losses prove both the necessity of compensation *and* the increased importance of non-monetary reasons and rewards.

To be sure, the relatively decreasing importance of money may be partly due to potential attrition. Women who are primarily interested in money may change their mind about becoming a surrogate once they learn more about the process and the risks. They may realize that the process often takes a lot longer than they had imagined, and they may understand that surrogates do not get paid before they are pregnant and receive very little money when they miscarry. Those who end up committing to surrogacy may increasingly value nonmonetary rewards as they build a closer relationship with their IPs, grieve over failures, and resolve to succeed in giving them a baby; these reevaluations are then reflected in their stories:

> When I saw on an agency website that you could get $20,000 I almost fell off my chair! . . . However, that was before I did any real investigating about surrogacy in depth, before I met my first IPs, before I was signed with the agency.

Once I met my first IPs, the whole money thing went right out the window. At that point, the money was the bonus. 2 years later . . . obviously I'm doing it for a lot more than the money—because I've been through A LOT with nothing to show for it—no baby, and no comp. And yet I keep going. For me, NOW, it's all about making a difference in someone's life. A chance to teach my kids to be selfless, and do for others. A chance to make the world a little tiny bit better. I want to experience that feeling of seeing new parents holding their baby for the first time. I certainly can't change the world—but I totally can make someone's life better by helping them create their family.

Sure, the money will still be great . . . but it's so much more than that. . . . by the time I got involved with surrogacy, it wasn't about the money anymore.

Money is a significant factor even as priorities change. Compensation is not only for the surrogate's pain and suffering but also for the hardships the whole family endures: "the money is a thank you to my family for putting up with something that is an inconvenience to them." Numerous threads elaborate the sacrifices the family, especially husbands, have to make. Patsy playfully observed that "my DH says that comp is for him for having to put up with a pregnant, hormonal lady for 9 months!" Children are affected, too. "You cannot really make up for the times when I couldn't pick up my kids, or couldn't play with them because I was throwing up, and my two-year old didn't understand why she couldn't sit on my lap," pointed out Sara, but "at least part of the comp paid for a trip to Disneyland."

Much like Sara above, SMO-ers often voluntarily disclose what they spend the comp on. However, they do not like it "when IPs or agencies ask what our plans for the comp are. Why does it matter?" Discussions show that women often use the comp to pay off family debts and student loans or on the down payment for a house. Another common practice is to save some of it for their children's college education, spend some on family vacation, usually to Disneyland, or a new truck or jeep for the husband. A few women joked about spending some of the comp from their last surrogacy on a tummy tuck, but I have not read threads in which women discussed actually having done this.

Whether surrogates spend any of the compensation on plastic surgery or not, these jokes are meant to underline both the bodily toll surrogacy takes and surrogates' right to spend the money the way they want to without anyone judging them. However, discus-

sions about this issue generally echo Ragoné's finding that surrogates do not spend the money on themselves or themselves alone.[19]
By using their compensation for family-related purposes such as
down payments, college savings, cars, and vacations, surrogates not
only acknowledge their family's contribution but affirm and sustain
the primacy of these relationships in the present and future. As
wives and mothers, they want to reward and benefit husbands and
children who made sacrifices, too. Money serves to assert the equality between the IPs' and the surrogate's family on the principle that
no one should only give and not receive.

In some cases, when after the birth IPs redefine the relationship as a terminable business relation, surrogates regret not having
charged more. After the birth, Lynn got "not a hug or nothing. . . .
I'm so frustrated of all of this I could just scream. . . . as soon as the
babies were born they got what they wanted." She was deeply hurt
because her IPs made "this whole arrangement into a business deal.
I now regret not asking for extras [extra fee for twin pregnancy]."
Her regret highlights the symbolic meaning of money in these, from
the surrogate's point of view intimate, relationships: when the relationship soured, the fantasy of charging "extras" meant a redefinition of the relationship to match the couple's treatment of her "as an
employee." There was an outpouring of sympathy on SMO. "They
should not have treated you like a business associate . . . surrogacy
is about love not money."

At first glance, these stories indicate an antagonism between
love and money. However, on closer scrutiny, they actually testify
to money's embeddedness in social relationships and to the social
understanding that the definition of the payment should match the
definition of the relationship.[20] From the surrogate's point of view
the payment did not make surrogacy a business deal as long as she
thought they had a loving and close relationship in which compensation benefits the surrogate and her family while her pregnancy
benefits the IPs. The IPs' subsequent insistence that they had paid
in full for services rendered meant the redefinition of the relationship. When a few surrogates redefined the relationship in revenge
and regretted not having charged more, fellow surrogates readily
understood that the issue had less to do with money than with
feelings of disappointment.

Redefinitions of altruism

Undoubtedly, the numerous discussions about money serve the
purpose of working out answers to social disapproval and criticism

and to accusations of commodification of babies and pregnancy. But refuting charges that surrogates are giving up their children for money no longer has the same urgency it did a decade ago. By revisiting issues of fees and reimbursements, surrogates are not simply rejecting charges of commodification but are making collective efforts to reconcile monetary rewards with altruism. Tiff expressed frustration: "I hate the schism and polarization that compensation is either altruistic or monetary." SMO-ers have learned to be less defensive and collectively assert their higher moral standard, which is a much more powerful repudiation of criticism.

There are times when surrogates on SMO directly take up the question of altruism. When Zelda, an intended mother, posted a bitter and accusatory comment about how surrogates "call themselves altruistic when they charge fees," many women retorted quite angrily that all surrogates want to help IPs; therefore, all surrogates are altruistic. They may not wish to help indiscriminately, however. "Why would a surrogate want to help someone who is obviously THAT mad and . . . wouldn't appreciate her emotionally and somewhat money-wise?" Surrogates who reacted to Zelda's post did not see altruism and remuneration as incompatible. However, they did see bitterness incompatible with valuation; Zelda was too angry and hostile to be able to properly value surrogates.

Posts like Zelda's provoke discussions of altruism; however, these conversations are also fueled by surrogates' own desire to define altruism and reconcile it with remuneration: "I don't have a set fee. . . . I would hate for a few thousand dollars to break apart a potentially great match. . . . there's still people out there that wouldn't do surrogacy for whatever reason for any amount of money, so fee or not, surrogates obviously have altruistic qualities." Or, as Evelyn explained, "For how much we put our bodies, minds, and hearts through there has to be a strong level of altruistic drive in each and every one of us surrogates. Unfortunately, we live in a world that doesn't understand altruism. They hear compensation and automatically assume 'Oh, she's in it for the $.' That is sad for them not us." SMO-ers may well be right about living "in a world that doesn't understand altruism." Feminist scholarship often views surrogates' desire to help infertile couples as a sign of "false consciousness."[21] More recent legal scholarship regards women as rational actors who set goals to pursue monetary gain but often assumes that surrogates use altruistic language as the socially acceptable gender rhetoric to veil financial interest.[22] What these scholars have in common is distrust of surrogates' altruistic goals.

Neither assumption captures surrogates' own meanings. SMO members collectively insist that surrogates should represent their own best interest and that compensation is well deserved; yet they also collectively define surrogacy as a selfless act of giving of which few women are capable.

Altruism is commonly defined as giving selflessly without any benefits. This definition does not resonate with surrogates any more than "false consciousness" or veiled financial interest does. In countless threads surrogates argue that they benefit in a variety of ways, including the "warm and fuzzy feelings" that come from helping others. Many women voiced doubts about whether it is even possible to be altruistic without feeling good about doing good. Toni called for a redefinition of altruism: "Even if we did this for absolutely nothing, the definition of altruism is that we did receive something in the end such as pleasure or happiness for having helped a couple become a family. . . . we still get something from it. The self-satisfaction of feeling humanly good inside and for having assisted God in a miracle. Either way, it's a win-win situation."

In this revealing post Toni directly challenges the contention that altruism is incompatible with rewards; monetary compensation, in her account, is not different from any other reward. Toni is making it clear that there is no such thing as getting nothing in return. Surrogates who have empathy for IPs benefit from surrogacy because they feel satisfaction at helping couples become parents. But Toni is saying more than this. She is elevating this helping behavior above the human scale even as she talks about "feeling humanly good"; in her account, surrogates are directly assisting divine miracles. Although not the most common framing on SMO, this direct linking of surrogacy to divine creation is not unusual.

Toni's conclusion that altruism benefits both the recipient and the giver resonates with surrogates on SMO. Shelly's post captured surrogates' puzzlement at why people find this reasoning problematic: "people are accusing the good doer of only doing [good] so as to gain something and not because it was the right thing to do. AMAZING how some people think!!!!" SMO-ers generally agree that doing the right thing makes them feel good, and thus they gain something that is valuable to them. They conclude that there is nothing to do about people who think that doing the right thing without any gain is the only definition of altruism. David Schmidtz's argument that an action is altruistic if it is motivated by genuine regard for others, even if there are other motivations, is a useful one for understanding surrogates' viewpoint.[23] As we have seen, surrogates often talk about mixed motivations and maintain that this diversity of motivations does not diminish their altruism.

But as much as SMO-ers challenge the narrow definition of altruism, they also emphasize that surrogacy involves a lot more than a kind heart that enjoys doing good. Lindsey explained the difference between the two kinds of altruistic giving she had experience with: "With something like being a bone marrow donor, I feel that the two weeks or so that I may have to invest will be worth it to save a life. I don't need monetary compensation. The feeling would be enough. But with surrogacy, there is just too much of an investment of everything, not to be compensated."

Audrey's view—"I personally feel like if you are a surro, you should do it out of the kindness of your heart"—received severe criticism. "This . . . is one of the biggest lines of crap ever and I get so tired of seeing it. Most people couldn't even do this for any amount of money unless they had it in their heart to do it," opined Helen. As much as surrogates themselves talk about the heart, they are very aware of the embodied nature of what they go through and are not shy to spell it out in discussions. As previous chapters have documented, surrogates chafe against rendering surrogacy as self-interested actions for monetary gain, but they also often find purely disinterested rhetoric somewhat phony and unrealistic.

Surrogates simultaneously call themselves altruistic and call certain talk "altruistic crap," and this is not a contradiction. They point out that their own sacrifices, no matter what comp they are getting, are proof of altruism, while others, who have no bodily experience of it, take altruism to mean uncompensated surrogacy. The two camps are thus not talking about the same thing.

Sacrifice and commensurability

Women who have bodily experience of sacrifice agree that there should be some recompense, even if it will never be commensurate with the time and effort spent on making IPs parents. Lynn compared surrogacy to art rather than paid work while also acknowledged its demands:

> Actually, with all the cycling and preparation that goes into it, it's more like a year of time. . . . When you average out the comp, it's not nearly enough in those terms. But, surrogacy isn't my JOB. It's my hobby if you will. It's something I do because I enjoy the end result—kind of like ceramics and painting.

Sophie's point exemplifies a common theme, the unrelenting physical and emotional requirements of surrogate pregnancy: "we can't just clock out so it is 24/7, being a surrogate affects our family even when we try the hardest. . . . All the energy you put into it, the worry you put into it, the love, the caring & dealing with others' emotions as well and trying to do it tactfully." She lists the intangible work that does not have a market price yet requires time and effort and involves costs.

Women frequently proclaim that surrogacy is an unceasing "24 hour, 7 days a week 'job'" and compute the "hourly wage," which is invariably way below minimum wage. They agree that with this "pay rate," surrogacy is certainly underpaid. They joke about how much they would make if they asked for the same hourly wage they receive in their job: "You have convinced me to go ahead and charge a comp and make it equal to my hourly wage. . . . I just hope they understand when I bill for over 200K . . . just kidding, of course."

Susanne's post below explains that payment does not turn surrogacy into a market transaction precisely because it is so little money. The computation of hourly wage is used as a rhetorical device to subvert the market logic and frame surrogacy as a gift:

> With the comp . . . I am getting $1.72 an hour . . . I am giving 100% of myself 24 hours a day, 7 days a week for about a year to give my awesome IPs a family. How could you NOT call it a gift?? Do you think someone would babysit your kids for 10 months 24 hours a day for free?? I even agreed to a lesser fee because I love my IPs. She didn't want me to take my ad down JUST IN CASE I'd get a better offer. I tell ya, I could NEVER get any better than my IPs!! EVER!! You can't find a babysitter for this much money . . . and I am giving my body, my food, my blood, pain, labor, injections, back pain, nausea, migraines, possible surgery, a needle in my spine, etc., etc., etc. . . . because I love my IPs.

Susanne juxtaposes getting considerably less than minimum wage with "giving 100%" of herself. Her post skillfully contrasts the market logic of "getting a better offer" with the logic of loyalty in personal relationships in which people are not shopping for better deals. Susanne's narrative foregrounds the incompatibility of these two types of accounting. Her definition of the relationship is one of love and intimacy, and she understands the transaction as a gift exchange. By talking about money, she is calling attention to the incommensurability of what she gives and what she gets.[24] "Defining something as incommensurate is a special form of valuing."[25]

Surrogates often indicate incommensurability by calculating hourly wage; they simultaneously employ and reject the market framework. Wage work is a market concept, yet no job is 24/7. Reiterating that surrogacy is an ongoing, constant doing that requires effort and includes hardship calls attention to the work behind surrogacy but simultaneously also makes the point that it is not like other jobs.[26] This kind of wage calculation exposes the absurdity of commensuration and at the same time calls attention to surrogates' ongoing commitment and contribution. Surrogates often characterize it as "work of pure love" or "a job of the heart," but it is not necessarily these affective features that distinguish surrogacy from market work, since people may love what they do and still consider it a job. The real difference lies in the embodied, unpredictable, and life-changing nature of pregnancy.

When surrogates insist on the incommensurability of the compensation they receive and the pregnancy they go through, they make a statement about the social worth and uniqueness of pregnancies and babies, whose value cannot be expressed in terms of some other, in this case, monetary, value. The extension of markets and commensuration into new spheres of life "may make incommensurable categories more meaningful, their defense more necessary."[27] The pricelessness of children is not a new idea; Zelizer documented how children became economically less useful but emotionally more valued, and consequently "priceless," in the nineteenth century.[28]

However, upholding and defending the incommensurability of babies is most pressing for those who carry them for others in fairly newly monetized practices. By insisting on incommensurability, surrogates also uphold their own uniqueness as human beings and maintain that they are not interchangeable wombs for rent. Neither do they think of IPs as baby buyers. The large sums many are willing to spend on having a baby is not perceived as its price; rather, it proves to surrogates that they are deserving parents who are willing to sacrifice for family.

These discussions set the groundwork for the characterization that all surrogates are compassionate and altruistic. When surrogates like Susanne call attention to the discrepancy between what they give and what they get, they underscore their empathy and love. Choice features prominently in these stories. When women talk about choosing to lower or forgo fees to accommodate their couple, they are making implicit claims about the relationship and themselves. If they give more than they receive, it is not because of ignorance, miscalculation, or coercion, they claim, but because they are givers who chose to help specific IPs. Even if a surrogate does not compromise on her fees, and no matter how much she is paid, surrogates explain, she is still altruistic because she willingly takes risks to benefit her couple.[29]

> A surrogate puts herself at risk for all of the physical and emotional lows . . . And how many of our sisters have given their all to IPs who were less than grateful? I understand that many IPs may also have suffered through their own traumas as well, but they did so in order to receive. . . . The surrogate does the same, but with a different emphasis. . . . she does so in order to give. I don't care if a surrogate asks for a million dollars, it does not make her any less of a person, any less compassionate, any less of a giver. Remember, the only IPs who would take her services are those who could afford it. I also don't buy the notion that if a surrogate refuses to lower her fee that she is "in it for the money" or "all business". It just means that she is wise enough to know what it is that she and her family needs, and she will not compromise on that issue. You don't have to be a doormat to be a good, compassionate and giving surrogate.

Surrogates both offer and resist sentimentalized accounts of helping people become parents. They emphasize their empathy and love for their IPs but passionately reject expectations that they should carry babies for others purely out of empathy. These reactions are not simply reiterations that surrogacy is emotionally, physically, and potentially even financially costly to the surrogate and her family but are part of the ongoing effort to define surrogacy as a mutually helping, reciprocal relationship between *two families*.

In countless posts surrogates reiterate that surrogacy is mutual gain as well as mutual help and highlight elements of reciprocity and equality with their IPs. They reject definitions of surrogacy as either direct exchange of money for services and babies or selfless, one-sided giving. But this has less to do with criticisms of commodification and more to do with surrogates' efforts to work out the meaning of surrogacy and match the transaction they engage in with their definition of the relationship with IPs. Reciprocal giving in these accounts is not the direct reciprocity of market relations. In keeping with surrogates' understanding of the practice as an intimate partnership in which families make sacrifices for one other, the monetary transaction is conceptualized as financial help to the surrogate and her family while she helps the IPs to become a family.

After years of discussing ambivalent thoughts about fees, surrogates increasingly easily accommodate the fact that they are compensated in this partnership. "I like to consider my comp a means for my family to accept the risks and complications of pregnancy, like not feeling well, or down time that I experience related with surrogacy. I don't see it as a paycheck." Linda agreed: "Pain and suffering comp is not 'income' and does not make me an employee." Payments are made in many social relationships without transforming them into relations of employment. Some payments, like child support, represent care and providing rather than exchange. "My son's father pays me child support, but I am not an employee raising his child. A baby is not a product, pregnancy is not a job, and I am not an employee."

Compensation and quality

The following discussion is a good example of how surrogates negotiate contradictions and how they decide what is and is not offensive about money matters. It illustrates the contextual and interactive nature of the emerging responses and resulting definitions. The debate below started with a post by Valerie, an intended mother:

> I guess my point was more for those who claim the money is not important. . . . If you are doing it for the money, like I said, that's your business just be open about it. Also, I was referring to people who claim surrogacy is not a job to them, but something they do simply out of the goodness of their heart. No-one freak out, I realize you can do it out of the goodness of your heart AND still accept comp. But there are a great number I have spoken to who say it's NOT a job and they do it solely because they LOVE pregnancy and want to help, money is not an issue. And then they hit me with 35k as a second surrogacy base with a whole bunch of extras.

Several surrogates patiently explained that, in fact, there is no contradiction between claiming that "money is not important" and asking for a significant amount in compensation:

> some surros say it not about the money and technically it may not be, but it IS for most of their family. So in one sense it's NOT what brought them to surrogacy but at the same time they do understand the money may make it easier for their family to accept when the surro is too sick to get out of bed, cook, clean, or just interact with her family. And being experienced you learn to really understand what it takes financially&emotionally to keep you and your family running smoothly WHILE helping another family.

These replies also serve as a reminder—to IPs and anyone else who may be reading these threads—that surrogates are not isolated single women but mothers and wives who live connected lives. Responses to Valerie's post were patient and respectful. Eve described how she felt guilty about the compensation amount her agency recommended, but her difficult twin pregnancy convinced her that she should ask not only for the "standard" compensation but for some important extras:

> My bladder has prolapsed, my ribs have separated and my hips were dislocating. Still, I delivered 2 healthy babies . . . proudly and smiled through it all because I was aware of the pain my IPs went through prior to their decision to find a surrogate. I never asked a fee for multiples and by the end of the pregnancy I finally knew WHY 99% of surrogates do. . . . I felt my pain was a small price to pay for my IPs' completed family and so I decided to be a GS again . . . and I decided to . . . charge [more].

The tone of the discussion changed somewhat when a former intended mother joined it, saying that it was wrong for repeat surrogates to ask for higher compensation:

> I don't agree with a surro raising their comp beyond the second surrogacy, just because they feel they are experienced. I think the more pregnancies you have, the higher the risk of complications and I don't feel like it warrants more money. I mean really I thought most surros were in this to help other couples and not for financial reasons, so if this is true then there really is no reason to keep going higher and higher. I have yet to see a golden uterus. I do feel an experienced surro should be compensated as such, but to me anything beyond $25k is ridiculous and greedy.

Most fellow surrogates loved Mary's following response:

> Just because we are doing it out of the goodness of our hearts we should accept a low comp? Sorry but no. I love my job . . . but would you tell your employer ". . . let's slash my salary by 20%." ??? No I don't think you would. Money we receive doesn't lessen or increase the love we have for what we are doing as surrogates. We deserve to be compensated because you know what? IT IS HARD . . . doing it for free + things going wrong = recipe for resentment. . . . It's BS that as a GS I have to spell any of this out for an IP. How anyone could be involved in the surrogacy world and not understand that we DESERVE comp is beyond me. If you don't want to pay 25k for a second timer then don't. By all means find a desperate surro willing to take $5K and let me know how that works out for you. . . . How many stories do we need to . . . hear of a low comp surro . . . being an all-around crappy person to realize that you are comping your

surrogate in a fair manner for a REASON? . . . What we walk away with when it's all said and done doesn't make it worth it: it is creating families that is worth it no matter if we ask for $12k or $35K. And really how dare anyone else presume to tell someone what their intentions are simply by looking at their comp.

Mary's reply is interesting not only because so many SMO-ers loved it. Normally, surrogates insist that carrying a baby is not a job and compensation is not at all like wages, but no one objected to Mary's comparisons, because her real argument was that love and payment are compatible. Strikingly, Mary is drawing a strong causal link between the quantity of money and the quality of the surrogate. On the surface, her image of the "desperate," ill-informed surrogate looks like the portrait many feminist critics have painted of women who carry babies for others. However, in Mary's account this "low-comp" woman is not the one who is exploited; rather, she is clearly a low-quality person who misleads and potentially exploits IPs. Thus Mary is making a very different point than feminist critics have. Good surrogates are quality people and quality is reflected in their self-valuation and thus compensation. Money expresses value as well as valuation.

"don't sell yourself short"

Bargaining and valuation
As the previous threads show, IPs sometimes appeal to surrogates' compassion, or remind them how they said they were not doing it for the money, in order to convince them to lower their fees. And although women often lower their fees out of empathy, they resent IPs' attempts at bargaining and understand them as a sign of lesser valuation. When IPs bargain, surrogates tend to respond by positively linking valuation and money, as Mary did above.

Negotiations about money have both practical and symbolic significance. Fees can reflect IPs' concern for their surrogate and also express surrogates' self-valuation. Nelly observed that proper self-valuation influences IPs' behavior: "people have a tendency to judge you and treat you based on the value you put on yourself." Laura wondered if low comp was correlated with low commitment and disrespect from IPs: "I have noticed though that several of the journeys that have ended up being really rocky were very low comp." Hillary agreed:

I hate to compare surrogacy to dog breeding, but my mother-in-law bred her Boston terrier and sold all but one, which she gave away. . . . to someone "compassionately" who couldn't really afford a dog . . . and the puppy was mistreated and miserable. Not saying this is the case with surrogacy, but I would believe it happens now and again. Sometimes it takes folks dishing out money on something to show they are serious about it.

Hillary's analogy may seem somewhat ambiguous; does she mean to say that IPs will mistreat the baby unless they paid for it? The context, however, points to a different interpretation. In SMO parlance, "compassionate" means uncompensated surrogacy; not being able to afford a dog thus works as an analogy for not being able to afford a surrogate. It is the surrogate, then, who is not valued or is mistreated because she did not cost the couple money. "Dishing out money" better guarantees both serious commitment to the journey and more appreciation for the surrogate.

This line of thought is not unusual on SMO and is interesting because it seems to contradict surrogates' claims that pregnancy and giving life are incommensurable with monetary payment. Surrogates routinely insist that money cannot replace appreciation. They find translating commitment and consideration into monetary terms troubling, even offensive, yet they also often use quantitative measures to evaluate the quality of the relationship. SMO discussions support the claim that "our desire to manage uncertainty, impose control, or secure legitimacy" produces new forms of commensuration, while we also associate rationality with commensurability.[30] Surrogates thus both challenge commensurability and devise ways of translating quality into quantity in their efforts to gain control of, legitimize, and manage the many uncertainties of the journey.

SMO-ers who are often uncomfortable with negotiating, yet do not want to be bargained down, get very frustrated at being called unsympathetic and "heartless" unless they lower their fees.

What gets me though is when IPs spend so much money on IVF, i mean tons, then when that fails and they turn to a surro . . . it's always the same thing . . . , we have already spent all our money. . . . the SM is the last resort and we get what they can pull together. And that really bothers me. . . . I'm just tired of feeling like we are nowhere as important as the IVF clinics. I'm sure they didn't ask them to come down on fees. . . . But if we as surros were to say that, we are heartless and don't care about others. . . . And i can't help that some IPs can't afford it. I can't afford all the things i want either. But

> i don't try to make others feel bad because of that. But because it's
> a baby we are talking about . . . it makes any talk of money almost
> forbidden in a way.

> In general, I'm not offended if a couple is up front about needing a
> lower than average fee. . . . I was however offended when one couple
> that I had talked to . . . wanted a lower fee "because we already have
> one child to take care of" but was telling me about their great family
> vacations [to Disney World] and huge house and such. I am glad they
> enjoy their vacations and their house and their car . . . but it's hard
> to feel sympathy for them.

The above posts make explicit comparisons between IPs' payment
to surrogate and the money they spent on IVF or a Disney World
vacation, indicating that for surrogates the problem is not the IPs'
lack of money; rather, the problem is their priorities, which reflect
their valuation.

When a newbie was concerned whether her IPs would be able
to pay for unforeseeable expenses in the future given that they
wanted her to lower her "very low comp," fellow surrogates not
only responded to her practical concern but addressed the implicit
question of valuation. They thought this was a red flag not simply
because of the potential financial risk; rather, they believed that the
IPs' attempt at bargaining was "inappropriate," "disrespectful," and
"offensive." "If you're already low comp . . . lowering it further sort
of makes you a clearance special with a blue light flashing over-
head," wrote Mimi. "Don't sell yourself short; this is a BIG deal and
you deserve adequate compensation," advised Jenn.

Money is not only a medium of payment but also a measurement
of appreciation and worth, a way to indicate as well as establish the
basic equality of lives in an otherwise unequal financial situation.
Women feel cheapened when IPs bargain: "You start to feel like an
employee. I haven't met a surrogate yet who wants her IPs to think
of her as nothing more than a womb for rent, or paid employee,
a bargain basement surro." IPs' unwillingness to pay what the
surrogate asks for could hurt her financially and is also hurtful
emotionally; to surrogates, it indicates a lack of consideration and
appreciation, especially since so many women go to great lengths
to save money for their IPs.

Annabelle, who had four children of her own and carried twins
for her previous IPs was willing to do an "average comp" surrogacy
for international IPs and "not charge for every little thing." However,
during the first face-to-face meeting with the prospective IFs she

realized they expected her to agree to a ten thousand–dollar all-inclusive fee:

> he said that he thought anything over 10K was "greedy baby selling."
> Now that's fine, they are entitled to their opinion. BUT . . . they
> thought that I should agree to do it for 10K with NO bedrest, child
> care, lost wages, maternity clothes, misc. expenses, babysitting for
> appointments etc. . . . Now I did NOT decide to become a surro out of
> greed (hello, there are WAY easier ways to make the same amount of
> $$ in a year with no hormones, emotions etc..!!) BUT how can I go
> and put my family at risk in that way when we aren't rich? It would
> be sooo unfair to my own babies if I were in the hospital for weeks,
> they were in full time daycare, and we went broke, risked losing our
> own home etc. for somebody I barely know . . . (and obviously this
> particular couple had their mind set that surros were all greedy from
> the beginning, so I think it would have been a miserable journey if
> I had agreed!!).

Annabelle was offended by their lack of respect, made even starker when the couple sent her pictures of their "huge mansion on the Mediterranean sea, very expensive cars, a big boat." The couple's failure to properly valuate her—and surrogates in general—also revealed their underlying and implicit assumption of inequality.[31] Annabelle understood that these IPs did not think of her and her family as equally valuable people; they did not care that she would be left "with no protection" for her children. "Why am I greedy for wanting to protect MY kids??" While surrogates on SMO often express some unease about fees, they also increasingly find giving in to IPs' bargaining attempts problematic.

Teman documented how Israeli surrogates were more afraid of being a "sucker," being duped into accepting less than their due, than about charging too much.[32] Not wanting to be a sucker holds true for US surrogates as well. SMO-ers point out that standing up for oneself is a moral responsibility. Not "selling oneself short" has nothing to do with selling oneself and everything to do with demanding to be valued.

> I believe that in *most* instances, when what was a beautiful rela-
> tionship comes to an end over what seems to be a money issue, it's
> really not the money at all—it's the principle behind the matter . . .
> it's the idea of feeling knocked down a rung or two on the list of IPs
> priorities that hurts so badly.

Money can express and symbolize devaluation as well as valuation, and not only when IPs bargain about fees. IPs' financial nitpicking already signals their lesser valuation; nonpayment, which happens as well, is a crystal clear sign of their lack of appreciation. IPs' failure to pay what they agreed to is understood as an act of betrayal; it hurts surrogates both financially and emotionally. Christie, who "put so much time and effort" into making her IPs parents, was "very torn"; she had tried not to mind that some payments were not forthcoming. "Because I love my IPs, I have let a lot of things slide financially, because really . . . it wasn't about the money to me . . . but now I just feel taken advantage of. . . . I am hurt." Fellow surrogates understood Christie's emotional response: "I'd feel betrayed, too, after doing all you did for them," offered Lori. "Intended parents who were as concerned about their surrogate as the surrogates were for them would remember [to pay] always and not just overlook payments as these IPs have done," wrote Carly.

Bidding and valuation

While surrogates resent being bargained down, cheated out of payments or reimbursements, and made to feel guilty about compensation, they also dislike being offered *more* money as an incentive to work with IPs; such offers look more like a bribe than appreciation. When an IM asked whether her husband was right to suggest that she should be "more aggressive" and offer more money to "try to win over" a surrogate who was also talking to another couple, all the responses were negative, as the following examples indicate:

> I would make it clear how much you want to work with someone even if she is talking with another couple. . . . That could be the difference between choosing you and someone else. I know if I had to choose between 2 couples I'd pick the one who really wanted me vs. someone who just offered me more money.

> I really don't think it would influence my decision either way. I wouldn't base my match on who would offer me more money . . . and I can't imagine the IPs truly being comfortable with it. I would think they would always wonder, "Did she work with us because we offered her more money?" And that's not the basis of the kind of surro-relationship I'd personally want to have!

Several women pointed out that offering more money was akin to bidding. Tasha spelled out why being "more aggressive" with money could be off-putting: "I personally have been offered as much as double the amount by one couple than another and I always choose with my heart on who to help. If anything, being offered more turns me off because I feel like someone is trying to 'buy me.'" Women suspect that IPs who offer to pay more assume that the surrogate is primarily interested in money, and this is as insulting as accusations of greed. Offering too much and too little are both offensive; both indicate that IPs think of surrogacy in a business framework and assume that the surrogate does, too.

Yet SMO-ers unanimously condemn classified ads in which IPs specifically look for surrogates "who are not in it for the money." This, however, is not inconsistent thinking; surrogates read such ads as implicit assumptions and tacit accusations. "I don't usually respond to ads that mention money at all. It just seems to cheapen the whole process. It is so much more than money." "I refuse to answer those kinds of ads, too. I find it offensive that anyone thinks surros are 'in it just for the money.' Where are these surros, anyway, because I sure as heck don't know anyone like that!" Ella thought IPs who seek a surrogate this way "will suffer for it. That sort of IP won't get any good replies to their ad because of that. Their loss. They ought to know better than to put an insult in their ad."

Others thought that mentioning money in a classified ad was appropriate when IPs wished to indicate their financial constraints without making assumptions or judgments about surrogates' motivation:

> I'll respond to ads that mention comp if it's along the lines of some-one who knows they need a surrogate with a comp in a specific range (i.e. We can only do a comp of $XXXX to $XXXX) but not one that acts like surros asking for a higher comp are money hungry. I think it's good to have the comp range up front because comp amounts do need to be taken into account when making the match.

"to keep the costs down"

Saving money for IPs

It is not IPs' attempts to find a less expensive solution that is offensive to surrogates; rather, it is the bargaining, the sense of entitlement, the negative assumptions about surrogates, the lack of valuation it represents, and the assumed inequality it conveys. In fact, as I indicated before, women very often want to save money for their IPs and start threads about cost-saving ideas. These discussions tend to proceed very differently from the ones about bargaining. In threads about bargaining the emphasis is on the unfairness: IPs complain about surrogates' fees but readily pay lawyers, agencies, clinics, and doctors. Cost-saving threads, on the other hand, included suggestions about "no-comp surro, no-comp egg donor, indy arrangement to save on agency fees."

All the IPs' savings would come from spending less money on the surrogate or on services they do not need because of the surrogate. Recommendations listed many possible savings, but none of them advocated finding low-fee or no-fee lawyers or doctors:

> consider using a TS instead of a GS. That will cut out needing an egg donor, won't need meds . . . no clinic retrieval fees or monitoring fee, fertilization fee, transfer fee . . . no meds for the GS. . . . If you use a TS you have the surrogate fee, do home insems and so no IUI [intrauterine insemination] fee, less risk of twins or triplets and so the chance of bed rest goes down. . . . Finding a SAHM [stay-at-home mother] as a surrogate will not have a need for lost wages if the surro is on bedrest. If the surro only has 1 child, that will cut down on child care costs . . . or if her children are older and don't need child-care . . . older children can also help more around the house. A surro who has her own insurance that is pretty good will cut costs as well.

SMO-ers tend to enthusiastically contribute to cost-saving threads, often with their own stories of saving money for their IPs. Mandy's angry response to the above post was thus an exception in such a thread, though it would have been a fitting reply in a thread about bargaining:

> no fee lawyer
> no fee RE
> no fee agency
> Insulting and improbable . . . really isn't it?
>   My children aren't here on this earth to play maid and *help more around the house* so that someone can have a baby. That's really rude to suggest. If I am on bedrest for YOUR baby then YOU pay for housekeeping. MY children are NOT unpaid help to pick up the slack . . .
>   How about IPs come clean my house when I am on bedrest and babysit my toddler for FREE since their baby is the reason I can't do it . . . might be a different story when THEY are asked to work for nothing.

She thought that such cost-saving IPs were "pretty selfish" and suggested they cut out "luxuries" like housekeepers, vacations, golf, beauty salons, and expensive cars. Her post was received with hostility: "Wow . . . what happened in your life to make you so bitter?" and "Did you forget to take your nice pill for the day? They are in the Bathroom on the third shelf behind your witching pills."

While a few surrogates ventured to say that there was some merit in Mandy's post because low-cost surrogacies may put a disproportionate and unfair burden on the surrogate, many others seconded the following response: "What an absolutely horrifying post. God help any IPs you have worked with or will work with in the future and any surros you may counsel." Many surrogates also agreed with this reply: "I'm sorry but saying that someone's child COULD help more around the house should not be insulting unless your child is totally pampered and doesn't lift a finger at all. WHAT is insulting however is assuming IPs are living the life of luxury." Several IMs posted furious retorts about how they had not gone on vacation for years. As it turns out, assumptions about IPs' "life of luxury" are just as insulting as are assumptions about surrogates "greediness." In this context, focus on money—IPs' "wealth" or surrogates' "greed"—symbolically equals lack of empathy, a callous disregard for others.

Cost saving and compassion

Just as discussions about lowering fees for IPs differ from ones about IPs' bargaining, so do threads about IPs' bargaining attempts differ from ones about cost-saving ideas on their behalf. The following exchange started with Nellie's post in a thread about saving money for IPs: "I honestly thought it was SELFISH to even suggest or even think that it is ok to ask someone to carry your child or donate their eggs to or for you for Free (or at a much lower fee) just so that they can cut costs." While posts like this are common and generate agreement in threads about bargaining, this is not the case in cost-saving discussions.

When Lillian opined that few educated surrogates would offer their eggs or wombs for free, surrogates responded quite angrily: "You do realize you are insulting a lot of intelligent, educated, COMPASSIONATE women here? Many have offered or done low cost surrogacies, are they stupid for being compassionate giving people?" There was no shortage of sarcastic answers, either: "Well, Ya' ll. Since ima lower comped surro, I musta been dropped on my head as a child 😁 because I tink I am un-edumacated! How dare I take less to help someone fulfill a dream? Oh, crap, my intelligence always resurfaces because my sarcasm comes out yet again. WHY does it out me???? DERNIT!!!"

These posts are a far cry from Mary's, quoted earlier, which explicitly associated low compensation with low quality. The above passages articulate that intelligence, knowledge, and compassion are not only compatible but also necessary characteristics of good surrogates. These are not the desperate and unreliable low-cost surrogates of Mary's post but responsible, informed, and caring low-cost surrogates. Discussions assert that saving money for IPs, even at some cost to oneself, is what compassionate and empathic surrogates willingly do. And because it is surrogates rather than IPs who initiate cost-saving strategies, valuation works out differently in this scenario. Saving money for IPs, as opposed to being bargained down by them, indicates surrogates' sensitivity rather than IPs' insensitivity. Surrogates who cut costs for their IPs are not "suckers."

There are always a few women whose stories of self-sacrifice go above and beyond the typical range:

> The major reason that all of my arrangements have been private [without an agency] is to keep the costs down for my IPs. I have done all the legwork, from finding doctors and setting up appointments to making sure the contract is complete. This does not mean that I feel entitled to raise my fee for the extra effort that I put into it. This is my third surrogacy, and I will have received less compensation for the three pregnancies than some of you receive for your first. . . . it fulfills FOR ME the reason I became a surrogate. It's not about raising the quality of life for my family. It's not about maintaining the quality of life for my family. Yes, pregnancy can be hard. My own pregnancies have been easy and uncomplicated and I expected my surrogate pregnancies to be the same. They haven't been, but I don't complain. . . . I really think you're kidding yourself when you talk about doing this out of love and compassion and still find it necessary to justify every extra cent you can get out of your IPs. In this case, call it what it is—a business arrangement.

Such competitively idealized self-presentations imply that doing more for less money is the hallmark of true compassion. But while we have seen that "greed" is symbolically opposed to compassion, less compensation is not automatically associated with more empathy. Surrogates often perceive the thinly veiled disrespect—what Goffman calls "ritual profanation"—in such posts and refuse to concede the point.[33] "I am bothered by the implication that those who . . . receive less are somehow 'better' surrogates than the rest of us." Most SMO-ers bristle at these "holier than thou" posts, and sometimes jokingly remark, "here we go again!" "What pisses me off to no end, is the judgmental, holier than thou, belittling comments that one person makes against another because of choices made."

SMO-ers thus emphasize and restore basic equality among surrogates; if no one is less of a surrogate for accepting compensation, no one is "better" just because she receives less money. These examples also show that surrogates, much like other people in all kinds of social situations, "must rely on others to complete the picture" they paint of themselves—"the part expressed by the individual's demeanor being no more significant than the part conveyed by others."[34] Self-worth and respectability are the products of "joint ceremonial labor" among surrogates on the boards, where claims for collective superiority are not unusual but assertions of individual superiority are not kindly received or readily validated.[35]

Experience and valuation

In surrogates' eyes, however, different amounts of compensation do not necessarily indicate value difference. Yet there is monetary value attached to status stratification according to "experience"; most experienced surrogates obtain higher compensation than newbies do. Stella was one of the many women who wondered why experience should matter: "I think if you want to claim the $ is for pain & suffering there is no reason to raise it." Some women agreed that if surrogates maintain that failed pregnancies are not their fault, they cannot really take credit for successful ones, either. Success, they claim, is not a question of experience since every pregnancy is a new situation. Most, however, listed reasons for raising the comp, although not necessarily the same reasons.

These divergent understandings about the connections between experience and compensation give us insights into the meaning of experience and the distinctions surrogates make between paid jobs and surrogacy. Experience was relevant for jobs, some women pointed out, but "the whole job experience thing doesn't make sense to me. The longer you are at a job the better you perform usually so of course your pay goes up. But having an experienced surro doesn't really mean anything." But some women found the concept relevant:

> After going through this, I'll be an experienced surro and will KNOW that my comp will go up should I ever choose to do this again, because the amount I chose this time was not near sufficient. I guess you could say I'm experienced enough to know that asking for more is in direct correlation to knowing exactly how much pain and suffering I've gone through. Some other surrogates had also underestimated the hardships due to lack of experience. Knowing what surrogacy involves informs decisions about whether to raise compensation for second and third journeys.

There were other interpretations of the meaning of experience. Lana defined "experience" as surrogacy-specific rather than
pregnancy-related expertise:

> I agree with an experienced surro deserving a higher comp because
> they have 'proven' that they can handle the meds, the stress, the
> scheduling, and giving up the baby, etc. So I think that a 2nd time
> surro could/should raise her comp a reasonable amount, but if that
> is your reasoning or justification for raising your fee, then there is
> no good reason to raise your comp with EACH additional journey. A
> surrogate is either experienced or not.

Others maintained that experience was a significant factor not
because of the skills or endurance women acquired but because
an experienced surrogate by definition had accumulated more
pregnancy-related bodily "wear and tear." She was risking more
with subsequent pregnancies; experience thus directly correlated
with more "pain and suffering." Debbie agreed: "I think the higher
comp for subsequent pregnancies is due to the proven fact that tells
us that each pregnancy increases your risks." Thus women who
found experience a good reason for raising one's comp argued that
more surrogacies both entailed more risk to the surrogate (more
"pain and suffering") and implied "proven" reliability, hence less
risk for IPs. None of these posts drew parallels to accumulated job-
related expertise in work environments.

These discussions crystallize two distinctive ways of thinking
about the connections between experience and money. On the one
hand, as many women point out, surrogacy is not a job, so "the
whole job experience thing doesn't make sense." Surrogates are
not "getting better" at pregnancy, and every pregnancy is different;
previous journeys do not have predictive value for subsequent ones.
On the other hand, women pointed out that experience "proves
that the surrogate is competent in everything involved with surrogacy." Experienced surrogates are able to provide IPs with "peace
of mind," and their experience may even translate into savings for
their couples because they can catch mistakes lawyers and agencies
may make.

> If I were to do this again and raise my fees it would be because I'm
> experienced, period. There is a level of trust (you'd hope) that an IP
> can have. . . . There isn't hand-holding and the need to be cautious
> at every step and wonder if the surrogate will know what to do. I
> know enough about cycling that I will question when things don't

look right, when I know I should have a protocol, and I'll know what to expect. I also have a more level-head about major issues like bleeds and bedrest, etc. So instead of panicking and my IPs having to "take care" of me, I can support them and remain unemotional and balanced. I understand the toll it takes on my family and me and I plan accordingly, instead of putting the IPs in a "what now" position. I could go on and on. . . . There is A LOT we learn through being surrogates that is invaluable.

Women also point out that experienced surrogates may not have to go through some of the screenings and may have contracts that only need some updating, which also saves money for IPs. Even though they may raise their compensation with subsequent journeys, surrogates claim that experience usually translates into savings for IPs.

A different perspective is exemplified in the following post: "I ask for whatever amount I feel is worth for me to carry someone's baby at that given time in my life. I have gotten 'regular fees', I have lowered my comp for friends and I have gotten high fees all depending on the situation." Wendy seconded this approach: "I like the perspective there. A big consideration is 'at any given time in my life'. As much as that can be a reason to raise, it can be a reason to lower." As stories indicate, women do lower their compensation and compromise on fees, often happily, for the "right couple"; subsequent journeys do not always mean higher compensation:

My base compensation has been different with each match. My very first match the comp was higher than any of my subsequent matches. . . . I felt like part of the reason was very personal. . . . I feel a big sense of guilt that I am being compensated for something that is like an art form for me. It comes from my heart, and I pour all of myself into it, and it's hard to put a price tag on that. And if I have IPs that don't have to worry about the money, then I won't have to either. But that's not what happened [in subsequent journeys], and I lowered my asking comp twice because . . . what mattered was what my heart said about the match. . . . So, my current match is quite a bit less than I asked, and more than I ever could have asked for a match to be. . . . And I feel really good about it, because they are the right match for me. But I still have to remind myself to hold a line, so I don't give the farm away, so to speak. Because the crazy thing about surrogacy is that we are mixing money and heart, and it's hard to reconcile those two.

This passage artfully juxtaposes "asking less" and having "more than I ever could have asked for." It also spells out a very common approach and thus dilemma: if what the "heart feels" is more important than money, but money practices also symbolize relationships and valuation, how does one figure out what to do and how much to compromise without compromising oneself and the relationship?

Surrogates' arguments about lowering fees emphasize the situational nature of their compensation, that is, money is situated in the context of the social relationship with IPs. If a match is a good one and IPs pay the compensation the surrogate asked for rather than bargain or look for someone else, then payment affirms the IPs' appreciation and the rightness of the match. If, however, IPs are not able to meet the surrogate's request but the match looks "right," the surrogate may lower her fees to accommodate the couple, thereby asserting that "love trumps money." SMO-ers maintain that there are no general rules or uniform standards precisely because to them surrogacy is ideally a unique and respectful arrangement between unique families.

"comp is really very personal"

Fairness and equality

From all accounts, money is not the only or main reason surrogates on SMO undertake journeys, often more than once. Money, however, is central; it represents, symbolizes, and makes calculations about many aspects of the relationship possible. Whether they emphasize that comp is well deserved or brainstorm about cost-saving ideas, surrogates underline the importance of fairness: "I feel that if I am going to better the life of a family then the life of my family should ALSO be bettered." Being bargained down implies that the surrogate was not informed, did not stand up for herself, and generally was not an equal partner. Taking advantage of IPs, on the other hand, unfairly tips the balance of power toward the surrogate. Neither scenario is conducive to a mutually helping relationship; neither fits the reciprocal win-win relationship that surrogates champion. Fairness is thus essential for what surrogates call a mutually beneficial journey.

However, there are a few different ways to interpret fairness. One line of argument is that surrogates should not be worse off after surrogacy than they had been before; it is only fair they should be able to "preserve the quality of life" they had prior to their journey.

As far as "appropriate extras" go, of course I feel that all medical is the responsibility of the IPs. Also lost wages. . . . A maternity clothing allowance is reasonable. Parking and gas reimbursement and travel are also reasonable. These are all expenses that a surrogate would not have if she were not pregnant or getting ready to become pregnant for a couple.

However, it is not always clear what expenses are the IPs' responsibilities. There are some expenses that women would not have incurred had they not been surrogates, yet they are not unambiguously the IPs' responsibility, either. The following examples are from a very long and heated debate thread that illuminates another definition of fairness. Kim was pregnant for her couple and had already agreed to do a "sibling project" for the same IFs about a year after the birth:

Would it be unreasonable for me to ask my IFs to pay for either my BCPs [birth control pills] or to have an IUD [intrauterine device] put in to prevent pregnancy between #1 & #2? I don't have insurance that covers either, so it will have to come out of my own pocket if I were to pay for them myself.

A few women thought it was worth asking the IFs, but many more were against it: "Yes, I think it's unreasonable to ask them to pay for your birth control. You have other options to an IUD, including male birth control. It's not their responsibility to make sure you don't get pregnant."

Most responses emphasized that since Kim chose to do the sibling project, it was her responsibility to make it happen: "if you're committing to do a sibling project then you need to do what is necessary to make sure you can fulfill that commitment." Fairness dictated this: "it is your choice to do another surrogacy, so I would think any costs you incur for that part of the decision making process are on you. Any costs directly related to the surrogacy journey itself are on the IPs." An IM seconded these opinions: "YOU are choosing to do another one in the future. So in order to fulfill your next dream, you need to make sure your body is ready. So YOU would be responsible. Just because the IPs are party to the surrogacy doesn't mean they get to foot the bill for everything. Nickel and diming IMO." Surrogates mostly agreed, although a few remarked that this IM was "yelling the YOU and it just comes off rude."

Ella, the voice of reason, explained, "just because you have to DO something for the surrogacy, does not mean your IPs should be responsible for paying for [it]." When Kim explained that she asked the question in the first place because she would not have her IUD removed within a year, and thus not incur extra cost if she were not doing surrogacy, some responses got hostile, asking her not to explain anymore: "you're making yourself look like a money grubbing uterus #hore."

"Money-grubbing" is the most offensive epithet on SMO, and "nickel and diming" intended parents is a pejorative term that frequently comes up in discussions. Once in a while a surrogate explicitly posts some provocative debate starter about how "some surros" charge for everything, "sucking their IPs dry," often using the thread as a platform to showcase their own selflessness: "As a human being, helping sometimes means sacrifice. . . . I guess I just don't understand how women can say that they are not in this for the money . . . but still are able to suck their IP's dry! ON PURPOSE!!!!"

Incendiary posts like this usually give rise to heated discussions. "Basically you just insulted pretty much all the surrogates on this board for accepting compensation for their surrogacies," read the first response. Sensibly, many women pointed out that if both parties agree to the fees, it cannot be called "sucking the IPs dry." Others got a bit defensive and emphasized how they do not ask for reimbursements they are entitled to in order to save money for their IPs. As much as surrogates routinely discuss the importance of fair compensation, they often shift the focus to sacrifice when their empathy and motivation are called into question: "I am def. not a person that is in this for the money and I don't intend on sucking my IPs dry. . . . I opted to not 'charge' for a lot of things and took the low end of everything that I possibly could, but I am very offended by this post."

Depending on how positions are formulated, replies can be helpful and informative or belligerent and hostile. Newbies sometimes get into trouble for wording the question in a way that suggests excessive interest in money. "What is the asking price for a sibling journey?" asked Emmeline. "Asking price for sibling journey~ I dunno kinda struck me wrong there," wrote Molly. "UMM MEE TOOO!!! it wasn't just you. . . . I don't have a PRICE for surrogacy. . . . I am COMPENSATED," Candy joined in the criticism. Emmeline then apologized profusely: "It was late and I was struggling to find the right words. I did go back a few times and erase the 'asking price' (I knew this wasn't it, but couldn't for the life of me come up with what I wanted to say). . . . COMPENSATION." She even promised to ask the moderators to take down her post and replace it with a properly worded one. She was promptly forgiven: "No need to worry. We all have those moments of brain freeze."

This and many similar posts testify to the importance women attach to such distinctions and the urgency with which they make them. Compensation is the term women agree on and use as appropriate for the surrogacy relationship. Words matter because they stand for different practices and different "relational packages," that is, variable connections among interpersonal ties, economic transactions, media for these transactions, and negotiated meanings.[36] The "relational packages" are clearly different in the above example of price versus compensation. The former evokes "baby selling"; the latter acknowledges the surrogate's and her family's sacrifice.

Sacrifice and fairness are not mutually exclusive. Patty pointed out that surrogates fit the definition of hero, that is, someone who goes beyond the "call of duty" to risk her life for someone else, and how this calls for reciprocity:

> I'm definitely a hero as are my fellow surrogates. We have all risked our lives for someone else. It's very hard to understand the surrogacy mindset without actually REALLY thinking about doing it. As a TS, you are giving a part of you to another couple to help them fulfill their dreams of being a parent. . . . As a GS, you face many invasive procedures, months of injections (some which may be harmful . . .), not to mention a higher risk of multiples. Surrogacy isn't something that someone wakes up one morning and looks in the classifieds and says, "What will I do for some extra cash today?" It's almost like a calling, if you will. It is a deep desire to help someone. . . . An ER doctor saving a life absolutely has a right to be compensated for his/her time. So do I. I deserve it and my family deserves it. If we lived in a world where money wasn't necessary than I'm sure I would feel differently. Giving and giving and not receiving just isn't healthy in my opinion. Everything in life should be give and take.

Jena explained the close connection between compensation and sacrifice, believing that understanding this connection could help people grasp the meaning of surrogacy:

> I don't think that you can fully separate the issues of comp and giving of yourself. To me they are inexorably connected. . . . The base comp is to cover the pain and suffering of pregnancy . . . she is assuming the risk. . . . However, to be TRULY compensated financially for every minute, hour, day, week and month of cycling, meds . . . test after test, then all of the pregnancy . . . the comp would be completely outrageous and not even remotely affordable for IPs. So yes, a lot of this is done out of love.

Unique relationships and average fees

Surrogates often say that talking about money is taboo, even though evidence counters this claim. Unease over money matters have noticeably subsided; surrogates have developed ways of talking about financial issues that incorporate the widely shared understanding that money is or could be one element of a complex motivational and valuational package. Money practices and meanings are firmly situated in the private relationship between surrogates and IPs: "People have all different types of arrangements. People even have different ideas about what 'reasonable' ranges are. It's a personal choice in terms of what is reasonable to you. Some people do it for nothing, others expect to be paid a higher than average compensation."

Over the years, women have debated and worked out what "reasonable compensation" means: "What do I need for me and my family? Not 'what did someone else get.' . . . comp really is very personal. . . . we need to make sure we ask for what is right for us and our IPs regardless of what someone else asked."

As I argued in Chapter 3, surrogates reject notions of a "standard fee" or "going rate" for compensation and insist that each case is different. Thus women symbolically insist on the uniqueness of each journey, each relationship, and each compensation amount. However, surrogates also discuss researching agency fees and SMO threads to see what the "average" is. Knowing what is "average" is consequential because asking for lower than average fees is a double-edged sword. It can signal selflessness and empathy but also jeopardize one's "worth." "If/when I do this again, I will ask for the average experienced surrogate fee, plus extras, which are on the low end. I'm worth that much, and it's what I feel comfortable with."

Knowing how much other surrogates ask for seems to inform decisions precisely because of the complex nature of valuation. "I based mine on market research, so to speak. I knew that if things went wrong, I would be upset if I got less than what others with my 'credentials' were getting. So after looking at agency websites on here, I knew what a typical first timer . . . was getting." Some women, like Donna, go further: "I ask for what I think I'm worth. I charged on the low end the first time, and found that to be a huge mistake. The second time I charged on the high end, and I think I deserved it." As much as women reassure one another that "every penny is richly earned" and warn against "selling yourself short," posts like Donna's invariably invite some sarcastic reactions. "I'm thinking that maybe I ought to be one of those surros that 'charge' $50K for my golden uterus . . . you know, one of those 'commercial' or 'professional' surrogates. Or was that the uterus whore? Can't keep them straight these days," wrote a surrogate who was "not comfortable" with her agency's suggestion to raise her fees the second time around.

Self-worth is both expressed and bolstered through money practices. Nevertheless, the connection between monetary and moral valuation is not a simple matter. Too much emphasis on money has the unfortunate connotation of professionalism and commercialism, implying that money is the only value and the only way to value. Too little insistence on monetary valuation, however, undermines SMO-ers claims that they are well-informed, rational, and intelligent women who, together with their families, deserve to be appreciated and valued. The relationship with IPs is negotiated and expressed in and shaped by money practices. However, value is not calculated in dollars alone. IPs' affection is a value that surrogates treasure; it defines surrogacy as an intimate relationship. As Gerald Clore pointed out, "Affect, like money, is a token of value."[37] Defining surrogacy this way also produces moral value because it affirms the prominence of sympathy, compassion, respect, care, and love against market calculation. To SMO-ers, surrogacy is women helping women, one family helping another.

Notes

1. Viviana A. Zelizer's work informs my analysis of the symbolic meaning of money in social relationships. See, e.g., "Payments and Social Ties," *Sociological Forum* 11 (1996): 481–95; *The Social Meaning of Money* (New York: Basic Books, 1994); and *The Purchase of Intimacy* (Princeton, NJ: Princeton University Press, 2005).
2. Zelizer, *Purchase of Intimacy*, 34.
3. Ibid., 41.
4. E.g., Gena Corea, *The Mother Machine: Reproductive Technology from Artificial Insemination to Artificial Wombs* (New York: Harper & Row, 1985); Martha A. Field, *Surrogate Motherhood* (Cambridge, MA: Harvard University Press, 1988), 28; Andrea Dworkin, *Right-Wing Women* (London: Women's Press, 1987), 181, 187, 188; Sara A. Ketchum, "Selling Babies and Selling Bodies," in *Feminist Perspectives in Medical Ethics*, ed. H. Bequaert Holmes and L.M. Purdy (Bloomington: Indiana University Press, 1992), 290.

5. Gilfoyle argued that "because the 'whore' was also a metaphor, commercial sex was transformed into a vehicle by which elites and middle classes articulated their social boundaries, problems, fears, agendas, and visions." This is equally true for commercial surrogacy; boundaries between family and market, as well as between "natural" and "artificial," and fears about the ever-increasing reach of money are being articulated through debates about surrogacy. Timothy J. Gilfoyle, "Prostitutes in History: From Parables of Pornography to Metaphors of Modernity," *American Historical Review* 104, no. 1 (1999): 138.

6. Georg Simmel, *The Philosophy of Money*, trans. Tom Bottomore and David Frisby (London: Routledge and Kegan Paul, 1978), 378.

7. In *Surrogate Motherhood: Conceptions in the Heart* (Boulder, CO: Westview, 1994), Heléna Ragoné argued that surrogates see surrogacy as part-time work. My data, however, show that surrogates use "work" in more ambiguous ways to indicate effort, active doings, and dedication and also the toll pregnancy takes on them. They never refer to surrogacy as part-time work and often say it is "24/7."

8. See James Carrier, *Gifts and Commodities: Exchange and Western Capitalism Since 1700* (New York: Routledge, 1995), 19–20

9. E.g., Kerri MacDonald, "Letting Go of a Baby, but Not the Emotions," *The New York Times*, 10 May 2013; Anemona Hartocollis, "And Baby Makes 3: In New York, a Push for Compensated Surrogacy," *The New York Times*, 19 February 2014.

10. Charlotte Allen, "Womb for Rent," *The Weekly Standard*, 7 October 2013, 29.

11. Susan Markens, "Interrogating Narratives about the Global Surrogacy Market," *The Scholar and Feminist Online* 9, nos. 1–2 (2011), http://sfonline.barnard.edu/reprotech/markens_01.htm.

12. Ragoné, *Surrogate Motherhood*, 58–59.

13. E.g., Mary L. Shanley, *Making Babies, Making Families* (Boston: Beacon, 2001); Barbara Katz Rothman, "Comment on Harrison: The Commodification of Motherhood," *Gender and Society* 1, no. 3 (1987): 312–16.

14. Ragoné also documented that many women were not aware that payment was involved when they first contacted an agency (*Surrogate Motherhood*, 57).

15. Sharmila Rudrappa, "India's Reproductive Assembly Line," *Contexts* 11, no. 2 (2012): 27.

16. Rene Almeling, *Sex Cells: The Medical Market for Eggs and Sperm* (Berkeley: University of California Press, 2010), 112–15.

17. Jennifer Haylett, "One Woman Helping Another: Egg Donation as a Case of Relational Work," *Politics and Society* 40, no. 2 (2012): 223–47.

18. Haylett found that egg donors similarly see the money spent on efforts to conceive as confirmation that the couple will be good parents (ibid.).

19. Ragoné, *Surrogate Motherhood*, 58.

20. Zelizer, "Payments and Social Ties"; Viviana A. Zelizer, "Monetization and Social Life," *Etnofoor* 13, no. 2 (2000): 5–15.

21. E.g., Judith A. Baer, *Ironic Freedom: Personal Choice, Public Policy, and the Paradox of Reform* (New York: Palgrave Macmillan, 2013), 95; Margaret Jane Radin, "Market-Inalienability," *Harvard Law Review* 100, no. 8 (1987): 1931. Some use less harsh terms; e.g., Field argued that surrogates cannot be viewed as making informed, meaningful choices (*Surrogate Motherhood,* 27). Similarly, Christine Overall claimed that surrogacy cannot be a free choice (*Ethics and Human Reproduction: A Feminist Analysis* [Boston: Allen and Unwin, 1987], 125).

22. E.g., Hugh V. McLachlan and Kim Swales, "Commercial Surrogate Motherhood and the Alleged Commodification of Children: A Defense of Legally Enforceable Contracts," *Law and Contemporary Problems* 72 (2009): 91–107; Richard A. Posner, "The Ethics and Economics of Enforcing Contracts of Surrogate Motherhood," *Journal of Contemporary Health Law and Policy* 5 (1989): 21; Kimberly D. Krawiec, "Altruism and Intermediation in the Market for Babies," *Washington and Lee Law Review* 66 (2009): 1–55.

23. David Schmidtz, "Reasons for Altruism," *Social Philosophy and Policy* 10, no. 1 (1993): 52–68.

24. Ragoné quotes surrogates who say that "the money wasn't enough to be pregnant for nine months" and understands such statements as both affirming the "pricelessness" of children and a way to define the children surrogates carry for the couple as a "gift" that cannot be fully compensated (*Surrogate Motherhood,* 58–59). This interpretation is close to mine; however, I take issue with Ragoné's characterization that surrogates "devalue the amount of money they receive" (ibid., 58). It is important to make a distinction between devaluation and incommensurability.

25. Wendy Nelson Espeland and Mitchell L. Stevens, "Commensuration as a Social Process," *Annual Review of Sociology* 24 (1998): 326.

26. Sharmila Rudrappa documented how Indian surrogates favorably compare surrogacy to factory work in "India's Reproductive Assembly Line." Amrita Pande argued that surrogacy is a "new type of reproductive labor," similar to other kind of care work ("Not an 'Angel', not a 'Whore': Surrogates as 'Dirty' Workers in India," *Indian Journal of Gender Studies* 16, no. 2 [2009]: 142). Kalindi Vora, however, found that many Indian surrogates "described the value and meaning of surrogacy as different from a job . . . and as apart from clinic and market discourses." They even maintain that carrying a child for others is "an extraordinary and even divine act." She also documents that some surrogates try to pressure their IPs for more money or other benefits; in this context, claims about the nonmarket nature of surrogacy may to some extent also serve the purpose of trying to benefit from gratitude ("Potential, Risk, and Return in Transnational Indian Gestational Surrogacy," *Current Anthropology* 54, no. S7 [2013]: S102).

27. Espeland and Stevens, "Commensuration," 327.

28. Viviana A. Zelizer, *Pricing the Priceless Child: The Changing Social Value of Children* (Princeton, NJ: Princeton University Press, 1985).

29. Surrogates intuit Kenneth J. Arrow's conclusion: "High risks do not have a monetary equivalent" ("Invaluable Goods," *Journal of Economic Literature* 35, no. 2 [1997]: 759).

30. Espeland and Stevens, "Commensuration," 316.

31. Expectations of equality are highly socially and culturally specific; e.g., Indian surrogates do not expect equality. Vora argues that in some cases they hope that IPs' appreciation will benefit them and their family in the future, and they try to establish a "reciprocal relationship modeled on that of patron and client" (Vora, "Potential, Risk, and Return," S102).

32. Elly Teman's explanation sounds right on target; it is a combination of differences in cultural understandings of money and also in the social organization of surrogacy in the two countries (*Birthing a Mother: The Surrogate Body and the Pregnant Self* [Berkeley: University of California Press, 2010], 208).

33. Erving Goffman, "The Nature of Deference and Demeanor," *American Anthropologist* 58, no. 3 (1956): 495.

34. Ibid., 493.

35. Ibid.

36. Viviana A. Zelizer, "How I Became a Relational Economic Sociologist and What Does That Mean?" *Politics & Society* 40, no. 2 (2012): 8.

37. Gerald L. Clore, "For Love or Money: Some Emotional Foundations of Rationality," *Chicago-Kent Law Review* 80, no. 3 (2005): 1162. Clore argues that if "we fall in love with an unworthy person or pledge loyalty to a demagogue, we are irrational, not because we have followed our emotions, but because we have acted on value that was not there" (1162–63).

Chapter 5

GIFT

This chapter is about all the tangible and intangible gifts surrogates and intended parents give and receive and the complex meanings and practices of gifting during the various phases of the journey. First, I explore surrogates' definition of the ethic of care and the morality of giving as well as their expectations of reciprocity. Second, I discuss their accounts of the material and immaterial gifts given and received and the meaning of these gifts as well as the problems they often entail. Third, I document they ways in which surrogates articulate the connections between gifts and sacrifice and work out the limits of giving.

"Giving the Gift of Life"

The ethic of care

Surrogates frequently describe themselves as "giving people"; they volunteer their time, give to charity, donate blood, and help neighbors, friends, and even strangers. "I do plan on doing another surrogacy I hope to do many more. As far as women liking to help people. I think that it is in our nature. I will go out of my way to help someone if I can."[1] "I have been on the bone marrow list for over 10 years and always thought that I would make someone's life better by donating my marrow, but I am so glad that I researched surrogacy and decided to do it. Some days it is all that keeps me going."[2] "I try to do what I can when I see the need because I know I have been helped out many times by caring people," is how some women explain their own giving in the context of a general ethic of care.

Judging from these self-characterizations and the regularity with which SMO-ers discuss giving and helping, it is clear that surrogates see themselves as people who weave ties of giving. Posts about giving provide a coherent context for women's stories of surrogacy and offer some insights into the morality SMO-ers embrace. This morality is reiterated in inspirational poems surrogates love to post:

> Time is not measured
>   by the years that you live
> But by the deeds that you do
>   and the joy that you give . . .
> If as long as we live,
>   we unselfishly give.

As experienced givers, surrogates are not oblivious to the dangers of giving: "Sometimes I think it could be one of my biggest downfalls as well though, because sometimes people expect it of you when you have helped them in the past." Fellow surrogates agreed: "Yep, it can be a downfall . . . but i guess if you have to have one . . . that's one to have! LOL" Surrogates are aware that their giving behavior is not always appreciated or reciprocated and is sometimes taken for granted, yet posts testify to an understanding that giving is still the right thing to do.

Generosity is highly valued on the boards. Giving is both a manifestation and a signal of generosity; the value of generosity supersedes the value of the return gift. With inspirational poems and stories of generosity, surrogates affirm that SMO is a community of generous givers rather than professional "carriers" or service providers. Both contract and giving involve a relationship of partnership between giver and recipient "in a single enterprise," albeit in different ways.[3]

The gift rhetoric

Elly Teman argued that Israeli surrogates start out as "business partners" and that the gift rhetoric emerges through the course of the pregnancy.[4] In the US context the language of gift is ubiquitous. In her work on US surrogacy, Helena Ragoné found the gift rhetoric to be more prevalent among traditional surrogates; on SMO, however, all surrogates use gifting language.[5] "Giving the gift of life" is a commonly used phrase, and it predates SMO, having been popularized by some surrogacy programs in the later 1980s and early 1990s.[6] Surrogates have embraced this term and infused it with rich and personal meanings. The "gift of life" forecloses interpretations of "baby selling" or "womb renting." The obligations inherent in gift practices and the enduring connections gift exchange creates represent the antithesis of market relations in modern societies, where a wide range of obligations are regulated by contract.

In the modern economic theory of "pure utility," things "are seen as antithetical to the person's true self," and there is a moral "separation of persons from things."[7] We can make better sense of surrogates' discussions of gift and sacrifice, as well as their distaste for a business relationship, if we take into account how the gift represents the opposite of pure utility by signifying obligations of a different type. The gift framework thus achieves complex goals; it opposes the utilitarian logic and reaffirms obligations and reciprocity in an ongoing relational mode. "We both gave gifts . . . in surrogacy, it's not a tit for a tat . . . we don't keep score," explained Naomi. Gift exchange and the links it fosters stand for moral obligations by moral actors.

The "gift of life" bests other gifts and is considered the "ultimate gift"; this rendering carries distinctive Christian associations of sacrifice. SMO-ers are in agreement that surrogacy involves sacrifice, although they have different ideas about what is appropriate and what may be excessive; I will return to this point later in the chapter. However, this still leaves the question of the gift unanswered. What exactly is the gift?

Ragoné concluded that "surrogates define the children they carry for couples as 'gift.'"[8] My findings, however, indicate that the surrogate's gift is not this simple. Traditional surrogates say they give "a piece of themselves" or a "part of their DNA" and fellow surrogates praise them for being such amazing, giving people. Similarly, Sue, a three-time GS said, "We are literally giving a part of ourselves and a little bit of [our] hearts whenever we do this that to me is such a fulfilling feeling and can be addictive." Also, gestational surrogates maintain that part of their gift is embodied endurance: "all the shots and medication," the occasional adverse reactions to hormones, the emotional and physical hardships of miscarriages, failed conceptions, and repeated transfers, and the sometimes lengthy waiting periods in between. When they are successful at achieving pregnancy, gestational surrogates carry multiples much more often than traditional surrogates do; they tend to have more difficult pregnancies, and sometimes are ordered to be on bed rest.[9] Surrogates who carry twins or triplets are also more likely to miscarry and go into premature labor. Even unproblematic pregnancies are monitored closely. "The pregnancies in my experience were routine, the level of monitoring was not. I am sure that most SMs would echo my sentiments." And they do: "my OB monitored it more closely because IVF does have a slightly higher risk for certain things, but mostly just because the pregnancy was just so darn important and took so much to achieve." Assisted technologies are associated with increased risks for surrogates: "There are all the risks of the meds, the risks of the procedures, the risks of a multi-fetal pregnancy, the increased risk of hypertensive disorders." In a somewhat dramatic vein, Sandra defined the gift she and other surrogates give: "I am offering the risk of my LIFE for people to have a child. That is the gift I offer."

All surrogates give of themselves even when they do not give a "piece of themselves." "How anyone could think I would or could carry someone else's children, keeping them safe and sound until their birth, and be doing it strictly as 'a business transaction', truly doesn't understand what it takes to give of yourself." Both traditional and gestational surrogates talk about "giving the gift of life," by which they mean both the process of achieving pregnancy and the pregnancy itself rather than the resulting baby.

A three-time GS described what many call "giving life to the dreams of our IPs" and "sharing the miracle":

> Sharing the exciting news that I was pregnant, going to the first ultrasound and seeing the tears of pure happiness when the parents saw the babies for the first time, hearing the IMs choke up on the phone when they could not make prenatal appointments so I called them on my cell and put it on speaker phone so they could hear the heart beat and know that everything was going well, having them put their hand on my belly and talk to their baby and getting so excited.

This post is a good example of some of the other gifts involved: the surrogate's happy news of pregnancy and reports of the appointments and allowing IPs to "share" the pregnancy and "of course the birth." Surrogates often want to know what they could do for their couple to facilitate such sharing. Katharina, a gestational surrogate, asked intended parents: "what would make YOU feel good?" One intended mother answered in length, calling her post "Lightbulb reply":

Pay attention to your gut as you interact with your IPs. And keep talking as openly as possible to them.

. . . Here are some things that my GS had done that have made me feel like an active part of the pregnancy process:

—We talk a lot (but that's part of our personalities).

—She shares about the pregnancy process physically (I asked)— morning sickness, headaches, level of fatigue, etc.

—She calls me with the FIRSTs: first time she threw up, first time she noticed her belly growing and chest increasing in size, first time she had a food craving, first time she noticed a food aversion, first time she had an aversion to a smell, etc.

—All of us have gone to ultrasounds.

—All of us have attended OB appointments.

—We've discussed labor/delivery some already . . .

—We've gone shopping: maternity & baby clothes.

—GS has given me several gifts for the baby/us as parents.

These details illuminate the many small, intimate, and ongoing gifts surrogates give to make IPs feel it is *their* pregnancy and to create the closeness and shared experience that makes for "amazing journeys." Even though this IM prefaced her list by saying "everybody's different," judging from discussions, many other IPs want exactly the same things to feel included.

Surrogates often post about doing everything in their power to enable IPs to attend the birth, sometimes agreeing to have labor induced. "Even if I had a bad relationship I can't imagine not being on top of things about delivery and doing everything I could possibly do on my part to give them a chance to be there. Anything less on the part of a surro would be selfish." At times they accommodate not only the couple but the grandparents-to-be as well. Some hospitals limit the number of people in the delivery room; surrogates are asked to choose IPs over husbands, who provided daily support throughout the pregnancy.[10] "Giving IPs hope"; taking risks; "growing the baby"; sharing the pregnancy in numerous ways to enable IPs to "feel" pregnant, be excited, and be present at the birth, sometimes even rooming with the surrogate after the delivery[11]—all these are the surrogate's gifts.

Even when women write about "giving the most precious gift, a baby," they also uniformly assert that the baby was the IPs' to begin with. If, as surrogates often say, "you cannot give away what was not yours to begin with," you cannot give what belonged to someone else as a gift, either. Thus, as Teman's findings also indicate, and contrary to Ragoné's conclusion, it is not the baby that is the gift.[12]

Rather, the baby is the embodiment of a long and often arduous process. It is the baby that makes another woman a mother and turns the couple into parents; it is the gift of parenthood surrogates wish to give.

Gift, reciprocity, and gratitude

Surrogates expect to see their IPs' happiness and excitement in return for the gift of parenthood. "Seeing the joy in the IPs' eyes" is such a frequently used phrase on the boards that it sounds hollow after a while—until a few poignant expressions make it sound real again. Angelina expressed this sentiment in a sad e-mail to me: "I wanted to see the joy through their eyes. I wanted to feel the excitement through their smiles. I guess now I never will. I had to give that up with my IF a long time ago but now to not get it from my IM is just terrible."[13]

SMO-ers understand surrogacy as a bond of reciprocity. Gifts, as Mauss's classic study tells us, engender obligations of giving and receiving, connecting people in a cycle of reciprocity.[14] Through reciprocal giving people exchange aspects of themselves since gifts, unlike commodities, are inalienable and carry the identity of the giver and the relationship between giver and recipient.[15] Gifts are freely given in that there is "no institutional monitoring of performance," unlike in contractual relations, but gifts give rise to "expectations and beliefs."[16] Gift relationships reproduce and reaffirm interdependence and link transactors in durable ways. Although gift relationships entail obligations, these obligations neither call for specific counter value nor can be discharged by giving: "fulfilling the obligation recreates it by reaffirming the relationship."[17]

Lack of reciprocation can be devastating, and surrogates sometimes chose to see it as ignorance: "To see after the fact so many IPs with the attitude 'She carried for us, we have no obligations towards her after' or NOT sending pictures whether there was a relationship during or one party chooses (like in my case) not to WANT that same type of relationship afterwards is just plain ignorant!" This post makes the implicit claim that even if there was no "relationship" during the pregnancy or the IPs chose not to want a relationship afterward, in a more profound sense the surrogacy *is* the relationship as well as the gift.

Marsha's post also indicates assumptions and expectations about obligations beyond the contractually specified ones: "[the IF] wanted no contact with me. . . . he emailed each month to make sure i got my check. Only came to one ultrasound. But was all by the book. Contract to the letter . . . No xmas card . . . NOTHING!!!!!!!!!!!!!!" Surrogacy, these posts imply, is not simply a contractual but also a gift relationship; IPs are recipients of gifts and gifts entail obligations. IPs cannot choose not to be obligated, although they may be ungrateful.

In a very rare instance of male participation in a discussion about the surrogate's gift, an intended father made the following comment:

> my point is that you don't really get that at first—or at least we didn't. . . . I think that for IPs who don't already have children, the sense of loss about not being able to . . . experience the pregnancy all the way can be pretty overwhelming. It may be hard for the IM to focus on what an amazing gift you're giving her.

Some IPs never acknowledge the "amazing gift." Angelina was disappointed when her IPs proved to be unappreciative; her account also indicates that she saw her gift as the pregnancy rather than the baby:

> my couple made me feel that I would be part of their family for doing this and that made me feel that they truly appreciated the gift I was giving. Once they changed it put a whole new spin on things. I now have to look at this as a "business deal" which is anything but fulfilling but it is all I have left. . . . Part of my reason for "choosing" them was that they could truly appreciate the gift . . .right out of the gate not once the child is born and the journey is over. I need my IPs support now but they refuse to give it.[18]

Many others found that the couple redefined the relationship following the birth. After sending Christmas presents to her surrogate twins, Marjorie received this "devastating e-mail" from her former IPs. "We are extremely grateful and appreciate your services. Our contract has been fulfilled, so there is no need for further communication. . . . Finally, please be advised, that there are no misconceptions regarding our 'personal relationship'. This has always been a business relationship and should not have been construed as anything more."

The expression of gratitude in the first sentence rings hollow once the fulfillment of the contract is evoked. Contractual relationships specify the conditions of the transaction as well as the compensation; gratitude is the recognition that monetary "payment does not eclipse the gift."[19] Gratitude is the acknowledgement not only of the gift but that the gift "cannot be returned."[20] Acknowledging this may be a burden on intended parents, although few articulate these sentiments. One intended father wrote that he and his wife did not want to "bow down" before their surrogate forever; many others indicated a desire for "closure."

It seems that many IPs are afraid of the "tyranny of the gift."[21] Thus, some IPs reconceptualize the gift as service. Tessa's intended father, whom she called "dear friend" while she was hospitalized during the surrogate pregnancy (Chapter 2), did not even pay lip service to gratitude, saying that he had "no reason to be appreciative." After all, Tessa "did not do anything" for them that she wasn't "paid to do." This was strictly a business transaction; they paid in full and had no reason to be grateful.

Surrogates see it differently. Gratitude is a central concept for organizing the surrogacy experience.[22] Although some gestational surrogates say that traditional surrogates give more since they give a "piece of themselves," women generally do not expect more gratitude in traditional surrogacy arrangements than in gestational ones. In response to a fellow surrogate's complaint that people assessed her traditional and gestational surrogacies differently, Barb succinctly pointed out the similarity: "You, honey, are creating a life and fulfilling some lifelong dreams for a lot of people!" SMO-ers articulate the same expectation: "In both cases [TS and GS] the IPs should be grateful for the life you helped give them." A hopeful IM wrote in a similar vein: "GS or TS the IPs should have the decency and respect to update the SM, if for no other reason [than] that she did carry these babies for 9 months and did deliver them into the world."

Surrogates and intended mothers both use the word "should," indicating a normative moral obligation. Fred Berger contended that we understand the moral obligation to show gratitude if the giving that benefited us was voluntary, was intentional, and involved sacrifice; gratitude is the appropriate feeling when people benefit us because they want to help us.[23]

Yet gratitude is not quite like an obligation; appropriate feelings either arise or do not arise. Gratitude is "a somewhat unusual 'duty'" because "having a duty to have certain feelings and attitudes is problematic."[24] Surrogacy is an intriguing case because it is guided by contract yet also understood as gift. "I have had such bad luck with finding grateful IPs in the past. I never felt like my IPs ever "owed" me anything though. . . . It breaks my heart how much surrogacy is like a business deal," wrote Emmy, clearly differentiating between gratitude and obligation. Another surrogate explained, "I don't want my IM to feel as [though] she owes me. . . . I want her to CHOOSE and WANT to keep in contact."

Thus, not surprisingly, surrogates express gratitude for the IPs' gratitude: "I appreciate every single time that my IM says 'Thank you' to me . . . not that I expect her to constantly be saying it, but it really makes me feel appreciated . . . I appreciate THAT!!" Lorraine wrote to me about how happy and lucky she felt with her IPs and also distinguished between contractual obligations and gratitude:

> they have been so much more generous than just what the contract says. They always say how grateful they are to have found me. . . . But I am so fortunate to have them as my IPs. . . . there are times that the beautiful dream and hopes turn into a nightmare . . . and I feel so fortunate that I have found the perfect couple to help. . . . As far as the future with us, I can see a lifetime relationship.[25]

Surrogates' desire for continued friendship is in keeping with their understanding of surrogacy as essentially a gift relationship. "Gift both grounds and symbolizes a moral relation."[26] It is generally understood that "our ideology of the gift has been constructed in antithesis to market exchange."[27] Simmel argued that only the first gift is freely given, after which the recipient is under obligation to "return the benefit."[28] Obligation, however, is a clumsy concept to describe the bond between the parties because it does not express the ongoing give-and-take that is neither free from obligation nor coerced.[29]

"Friendship" is a better term for this uncoerced social relationship that "runs beyond specific obligations" and in which trust is central.[30] Gratitude involves beliefs, feelings, and attitudes; it requires certain "forms of behavior in addition to verbal expression."[31] These concepts are mirrored in surrogates' expectations for the relationship with their IPs. "I wanted and needed to be FRIENDS with the IPs and to have a relationship that would last," wrote a surrogate who felt excluded by her IPs. Women want trust, friendship, appreciation, gratitude, and sincerity. "I need a couple that is genuine when they say that they want to be friends forever."

The empathy paradox

However, surrogates' commitment to understanding and empathy creates a bit of a conundrum for them, as countless SMO discussions about IPs' obligations and gratitude indicate. Surrogates often find that the empathy they encourage and applaud on SMO works against their expectations of friendship and reciprocity. As I argued before, empathy prompts women to consider how IPs' traumatic experiences with infertility and pregnancy loss have dire long-term consequences, such as an inability to trust. Melanie, like many others, wrote about wanting to understand IPs:

> I can only IMAGINE what it must be like to have to trust someone else with your most precious cargo. I really can't even fathom it but I can be empathetic and when things got confusing for me or there were possible misunderstandings, I would just say to myself, what if it were ME in that position? That helped a lot.

Sue, who carried eight surrogate babies, explained: "On every journey, I've had an IM that was extremely guarded. Guarded in a way that infertility makes you." However, I never read a post that associated the IPs' trauma of infertility with an increased ability to empathize with others in difficult situations. It appears that surrogates have no such expectations for IPs. But in private some women do wonder about the empathy deficit: "I believe that people many times expect from others what they themselves are willing to give. I think this becomes a disheartening problem for surrogates. We expect that IPs have the same caring and compassionate attitude as we do."[32] In her e-mail to me, Ava added: "Shouldn't disappointment make people more compassionate?"

Yet surrogates on the boards repeatedly remind one another to be patient with couples. "I have vast amounts of respect for IPs for the hell most of them have gone through, and I try to be empathetic of the journey that has led them to surrogacy. After all that emotion, how can you really expect anyone to *know* how they are going to feel?"[33] Surrogates encourage one another to "give IPs time." In the following post, one surrogate outlined her strategy after not receiving photographs following the birth: "I am going to give them about another two weeks. If I don't hear anything from them by then, I will call and see what's up. I've been trying not to be meddlesome or a nuisance and to give them space, but I need pictures. Darned it. lol." Posts like this—considerate and devoid of self-pity—are always met with approval. Giving the gift of life thus entails other gifts—of space, time, patience, and continued compassion.

In order to generate the empathy they need to be patient and forgiving, surrogates repeatedly asked IPs to tell their stories on the board. They wanted to hear how intended mothers feel about another woman carrying her child with the stated purpose of becoming better informed. One such thread was started by Myrna, who had eight journeys and only one successful surrogacy. She wanted IMs to write about their "true feelings" so that surrogates, whom she consistently called carriers, would understand:[34]

> I believe that if a carrier knew how this news [the surrogate's pregnancy] affected her IM, or how her IM got thru the day knowing her everything rested within another woman's body it would definitely give her the ability to understand. . . . some carriers have said that their IM seemed distant {for a lack of a better word} during the pregnancy. Maybe the carrier felt as if she wasn't important to her IPs. If all she and her family were sacrificing for another went unnoticed. I believe these thoughts and feelings may all go back to the ability to understand. . . . So this is why I ask for IMs to please share with us, enlighten us. We need to know your honest thoughts and feelings. You will see plenty of threads made by a carrier expressing her feelings and thoughts of the whole process of surrogacy, but none from the woman who will soon be called "Mother."

This demonstration of unmitigated sympathy was welcomed by both surrogates and IMs and prompted some intended mothers to tell their stories of anger, jealousy, pain, and worry:

> every time I see a pregnant woman, or a newborn, I still get an overwhelming sadness, and am reminded of the emptiness that's inside. DH and I have started searching for a GS. . . . It is an uneasy and guarded feeling that we have because so much has already been taken away. We are scared of another failure, and don't want to get our hopes up too high. And just to be honest, another feeling I have is worry. Worry that someone else might not take as good of care of my unborn baby, as I would.

> I was guarding a pain that was so deep, I repressed it most times. . . . Yet, I was always so grateful for the prospect of someone willing to give completely and willingly of their very flesh and blood (we did TS) to make all of my dreams come true. I have to admit that I was so guarded, that I didn't truly enjoy the pregnancy part . . . . had practically convinced myself that either our TS would not be able to surrender the baby or it would turn out to not be dh's child . . . to me nothing compares to two couples coming together with so much mutual love and respect and supporting the creation of a child that has been so wanted for so long. Anybody (almost) can have sex and make a baby, but the process of surrogacy is so life affirming, I think if we all had to go through it there would be far fewer unwanted children in the world.

Surrogates responded with warm sympathy, especially when the concerns IMs expressed were dwarfed by gratitude and the conclusion that surrogacy is superior to other forms of childbearing. They sympathized when an IM who responded to Myrna's call for stories said that adopting "just didn't sit well with" her. A newbie was one of the many surrogates who were grateful: "I just want to thank all the IMs who shared their feelings. It made me open my eyes as to why some IPs distance themselves through the pregnancy. . . . Again thanks from the bottom of my heart!!!!" Surrogates, who in different threads find intimations of dishonesty—that they will keep the baby or not honor their promise to refrain from having sex while trying to get pregnant for the IPs—infuriating, responded to these IMs' confessions with compassion and a renewed sense of purpose. "My heart goes out to you all, I sense your guarded feelings and want you to know that we love what we do as surrogates. The majority of us come here to 'talk' because we love what we do."

However, being patient with and sympathetic to "guarded" and sometimes even suspicious IPs is not easy, given surrogates' expectation of appreciation for the hardships they go through. However, highlighting one's sacrifice risks appearing self-interested and self-absorbed. Thus, in discussions women emphasize each other's contribution, or surrogates' contribution in general, rather than their own. They are more comfortable demanding appreciation and gratitude for each other than for themselves. The following passage is a good example of outrage on behalf of all wronged surrogates rather than on her own behalf, even though the personal hurt clearly comes through:

> I just want to say, so many times people are willing to make sacrifices for a relationship, they are willing to work for their success. Seems like that is NOT the case with a LOT of IPs and surrogates. IPs think they can just turn it into a business relationship when it gets hard or difficult to make it work. HOW SELFISH!! HOW IMMATURE AND HOW RUDE!!! In case these IPs forget, if it was not for us, they would not have these babies in their lives. . . . I am saying we are WORTH the extra effort and time. . . . If these women are jealous or insecure then they should be woman enough to say so. I think we as surrogates could understand that and try to help them in this situation.

Even though the post begins with an evenhanded disparagement of both couples and surrogates who are not willing to sacrifice, soon the indignation is directed only at "selfish" IPs.

In another thread, Louise started her post by expressing doubt about her IPs' intentions of continued contact: "I don't know if they will follow up on their promises." She then quickly turned to sympathetically supporting Miranda, whose IPs had not been in contact with her since the birth nine months earlier and whose gifts to her surrogate babies were not acknowledged:

> I feel so horrible for you, I wish I was right there to hug you!!! I can't believe that people can be so cruel and heartless. . . . They must have some serious self-esteem issues going on, I guess if you buy the babies a present you must want to steal them from their parents??!!?? WTF???!!!! Talk about ungrateful.

Some surrogates advocate a somewhat different solution to the empathy paradox, one that does not pit having empathy against expecting appreciation. In this spirit, Alicia encouraged fellow surrogates to see things from the IPs' perspective while holding on to the idea that IPs are always grateful:

> I try to focus on the IPs all that they have given up in this process. How they have had to share their joys and sorrows with a third person. To me, the birth of my children has always been a very intimate . . . moment between my husband and I. I can't imagine having to share those with anyone. Our IPs unfortunately do. You will find that the joy and excitement in their faces when they see their baby being born will make the whole journey worth it. Whether or not there is a relationship in the future or not. They will always be thankful to you, they just may want to be "normal" parents without having to feel the need to "check in."

It is a seductive idea that intended parents will be grateful forever, even if they do not stay in contact. Intended mothers support this idea:

> I have been on SMO for a long time and have heard lots of bad stories. . . . Even though they [IPs] may not express to you how thankful they are. . . . [I] know they are. They may have bad feelings or something but they will not forget you. I hope one day they will send you an update and pictures, at least, and hopefully thank you for all you have given them.

IPs' gratitude thus becomes an "incorrigible proposition"; it cannot be proven wrong even if IPs do not stay in touch because not staying in touch can be explained as inability to express—rather than to feel—gratitude.[35] Therefore, IPs' cutting ties does not disprove the proposition that they "will always be thankful." In a very few instances surrogates reported that their former IPs contacted them after years of silence, and the news served as confirmation of the enduring nature of gratitude.

These instances of renewed contact are understood as apology for the wrong of cutting ties. IPs' failure to provide contractually promised updates constitutes breach of contract, but surrogates almost never seek legal remedy. They see IPs' behavior as a moral rather than legal issue; the gift of life should create the kind of personal relationships in which the couple would sincerely want to stay in touch. Stories of renewed contact initiated by IPs powerfully stand for the restoration of moral balance and of an "equity of regard" that women wish for even as they are frequently ambivalent and conflicted about expectations of reciprocity and friendship.[36]

The only times when surrogates find it easy to underscore their sacrifice and gift is in response to blatantly accusatory posts by prospective or actual intended mothers and "holier than thou" surrogates.[37] The following proved to be an inflammatory outburst by a woman who was looking for a surrogate after she lost a pregnancy and her ability to carry again:

> Where is the love? . . . I would never in my wildest dreams ever have believed that in a place like this [SMO], where hopefully new life is created, would there be so many cold & seemingly heartless people. Are all surrogates like this? . . . Do you think it's fair to say it's up to the surrogate how much contact she has with the IPs? . . . Do any of you have any idea how hard it is to LET another woman carry YOUR baby? The way most of you talk it's like you are doing us poor IPs the biggest favor, and we should be grateful, and do whatever you say. But you are being paid $30 000 aren't you?

Although surrogates confess to get "teary eyed" upon reading intended mothers' confessions of their true feelings, contemplating "how hard it is to let another women carry your baby," no one shed tears for this woman. While in many other threads surrogates frame IPs' choice of surrogacy as a need and sympathize with IMs with whom adoption "didn't sit well," replies pointed out that this IM *chose* surrogacy rather than adoption.[38] Provoked by the hostility of the original post, most responses were uncharacteristically severe:

> My IPs and I agreed on how much contact and they outright lied!! I have received NO contact. I don't know why IPs feel so threatened that we want your child when as you say, we can have them for free and with the ones we love. . . . I can only imagine how hard it is to have to let someone else carry your child, BUT that is your choice. There is always adoption, YOU chose this route. . . . Why is it so hard for IPs to care about their surro, treat them with respect, and feel that they deserve this fee.

I understand that $30,000 . . . seems like a lot. . . . However, I keep seeing a common theme among posters like you—it's this sense of entitlement, and I just don't understand it. Do you honestly think that we, as SMs, owe it to you to carry your child? . . . If you are looking for someone who wants to carry your child out of love— someone who asks nothing more than your gratitude in return, then you should turn to someone who is already emotionally invested in your happiness, like a family member or a friend. I just don't think it's right to berate other women, women you have never even met, for not giving you what you want. Nobody owes it to you.

Lynn did not mince her words, either, directly calling attention to her own sacrifice and the respect she and all other surrogates deserve, even criticizing those who responded less harshly:

I don't owe you or any other IM a child. I do what I do because I love doing it. And thank the good Lord I have been blessed with IPs that have appreciated the sacrifices I have made to be their surrogate. And not a disrespectful, bitter, snob!! . . . This woman . . . didn't come here for support or information, she came here to berate surrogates. Since when did becoming a surrogate mean you can't have any balls and stand up for yourselves??!!

In instances of "surro-bashing," SMO-ers exhibit no collective sense of obligation to be sympathetic and forgiving. Surrogates find it easier to forcefully insist on respect and appreciation when they are criticized and berated. The above incensed responses confirm the shared contention that surrogates do not owe anyone a baby and their willingness to carry for someone else is the first gift, the one freely given. Ideally, their gift engenders a gift relationship in which both parties appreciate what they receive. Surrogates' empathy, the nurturing of the pregnancy and dealing with discomfort, the determination it takes to complete a journey—these are all gifts, and not just to the IPs. Bringing children into the world, Marianna explained, means making a larger contribution.

For me, it's about making a contribution to this world that's bigger than myself, bigger than just my family and bigger than just my own interests. I wanted to take a gift I had been given, my fertility, and share it with others. I did this because I have always wanted to change the world, and with each new life I help usher into it, the world changes again forever. . . . Because there is nothing in this world we treasure more than our children, and the many ways they enrich our lives, and I wanted to help as many people as I could to experience that. . . . Because God placed a calling on my heart

greater than any other that drew me to this world of surrogacy. . . .
Not everyone can do it, and not everyone should do it, but those who
have been called upon would have to deny a huge piece of ourselves
to NOT do it.

Rachel's post effectively combines the private and public "gift";
she is helping both her couple and the world by birthing a child for
good people. "I can't do anything about evil, stupid, or incompetent
people reproducing, but I can counter the effect a bit by helping my
IPs add to the population." US surrogates always foreground family,
even when they are expressing a wish to make the world a better
place.

This stance is best examined in comparative perspective. Israeli
surrogates emphasize their public sacrifice; producing Jewish Israelis is understood as a mission that serves the country. Israeli surrogates want to give the gift of parenthood to couples who yearn
for a child, but service to the country is closely associated with this
private act of giving.[39] US surrogates use a predominantly private
and quasi-religious language: love, sacrifice, and giving are invoked
in the context of the relationship with the couple, not the country
or the nation. Surrogates in the United States build families, one at
a time, and these families add up to a better society. This imagery
is consistent with the American conceptualization of family as the
building block of society.

The Christian imagery is omnipresent. Surrogates often talk
about "being called." "I feel the Lord called me to do this and as
many times as I have tried to walk away he has other plans for
me so I have stopped saying this is my last one cause I just don't
know," wrote Trina, a four-time surrogate at the time, who went
on to carry for two more couples. Not everyone uses such explicitly
religious language: "I'm not a religious/spiritual person, but I too
feel like this is just something I'm supposed to do. I am just meant
to carry a child for someone, and make them parents." In numerous
posts women express both a sense of agency and a diffuse sense
of obligation: "I continue to do it because I would feel selfish for
not. As long as my health is not in serious jeopardy by becoming
pregnant and I can get my family to support me I will continue to
carry for someone else because I can and it would feel selfish to not
share that gift."

The following is an example of the most common expression
of motivation: "I want to give this gift to someone, and I want to
help someone who is otherwise unable to have the most fabulous,

important, rewarding thing a human can have: a child." Surrogates believe they are fulfilling a very important social task, the repro-duction of the ties of parenthood and family.[40] They are often very invested in "nurturing parents" and seeing them bond with the baby. Surrogates wish to transform couples into parents: "I wanted to be able to give the gift of parenthood to another couple and I did that. . . . I am willing to give whatever it takes to help another couple have a child."

"By being a surromom I am . . . giving life to the dreams of our IPs," is a concise articulation of a common sentiment. "I was aware of just how many people there are in the world who cannot be parents without someone else's help. While I was pregnant I had a few people ask me if I would consider helping them next and I knew I was not done helping. I could not be done helping." Being needed and able to "help" in such a life-altering event as having a child gives surrogates a sense of mission and importance that surpasses what other people, even helpful people, do.

At times surrogates have so much empathy for IPs that they are more eager to start the process than the IPs are. Linda, a TS, was not sure how to deal with her IPs' lack of enthusiasm:

> I must say that my IF is somewhat standoffish and gets very nervous about this whole surrogacy thing. . . . I do believe he wants a baby but I also believe he is doing this for his wife also. We cycled once in Oct., and then Nov. and Dec. was cancelled . . . said he didn't want to take me away from my Thanksgiving and we would just cycle next month. . . . But my IF again cancelled insems . . . I already told them for Nov., that missing Thanksgiving isn't a big deal to me . . . I told them again, that it wouldn't be interfering with Christmas. . . . I want to address this issue without hurting anyone's feelings, nor do I want to push insems on my IPs.[41]

Linda added: "I felt like I wasn't being taken seriously enough and this hurt my feelings." She did not see her intended father's rescheduling of insemination dates as considerate actions; rather, she understood them as delaying tactics, and so did fellow sur-rogates: "I really agree with everyone . . . I think this IF is just delaying due to embarrassment and just not 'ready.'"[42] The following reply reflects quite a few women's experience: "I was more excited about them becoming parents than they were." Fellow surrogates advised Linda to "move on," given that her IPs were less than dedi-cated: "We do put so much of ourselves into carrying for another. Cycling doesn't wait for The Holidays to be over, or for us to watch the Superbowl. We know that we may need to make a few sacrifices to make this work for our IPs and that is why we are so dedicated."

"love to give gifts"

Tangible and intangible gifts

In happy surrogacy arrangements, gratitude and gifts flow in both directions. Beyond the intangible gifts of trust, respect, and friendship, IPs give various material gifts, such as store and restaurant gift cards, flowers and gift baskets, lotions and soap; they also sometimes pay for housekeepers, massages, and other spa services.[43] Intended parents sometimes give toys to the surrogate's children or pay for a vacation or trip to Disney World for the surrogate's family.

IPs also give jewelry, especially at birth, with either the baby's birth stone or some other symbolic design, such as interconnected hearts. The heart motif was common in the jewelry gifts Israeli IPs gave their surrogate, but I did not find that the jewelry gifts predominantly memorialized the surrogate-intended mother relationship that Teman documented.[44] My data indicate that hearts and the baby's birthstone symbolize both the life and the relationships that were created by surrogacy. Angel designs are common, too, symbolizing the surrogate's selfless giving. The central symbolism is the same, though: jewelry is precious, thus a fitting gift for the surrogate's precious gift of life.

Surrogates almost always disclaim ever wanting or expecting presents. However, they enthusiastically correspond about the gifts, both tangible and intangible, they want to give to the intended parents. In countless threads surrogates weigh in on the importance of giving over receiving. Unlike Israeli surrogates, who expect their IPs to be generous and pick up the tab even when they are not contractually obligated to, SMO-ers are often uneasy about accepting such gifts.[45]

US surrogates seem quite conflicted about IPs' gestures of giving; they love to be appreciated and cared for yet are uncomfortable with taking IPs for granted. Expecting IPs to pay for meals when they go out, for example, strikes surrogates as "greedy" and "taking advantage of IPs" and is often problematized on the message boards: "you do eat even when your IPs are not around so why should they pay for your meal when you go out together?" Surrogates agree, though, that going out with IPs is a great way to enjoy each other's company and having time together is enough of a gift.

SMO-ers often disclaim interest in material gifts, preferring to be included in social events and treated as an equal. When an intended mother asked what would be a good present for the surrogate at the baby shower, many replies pointed out that "just being there and sharing that special day with you is a wonderful gift in itself."[46] They also pointed out that the baby shower is not about the surrogate but "all about the baby and helping you become a mommy."

Gifts are much less often discussed on the "Parents via Surrogacy" forum. When one IM, who was "not usually a big gift giver," asked whether she should bring anything to the "first date" with the surrogate and her family, a few IMs suggested somewhat generic gifts, such as flowers and sparkling lemonade for the surrogate's children. The relative paucity of discussions about gifts on this forum indicates an imbalance between IPs' and surrogates' preoccupation with giving. Intended mothers occasionally post questions on the general surrogacy forum about what to give to their surrogate; most of these queries are about gifts for after the birth.

Surrogates usually suggest some favorites, like a heart-shaped pendant or a relaxing massage paid for by the couple, but there is an unmistakable preference for gifts of contact and updates: "The best thing that my first IPs did for me and still do is continue to send photos (she's 3 years old now) and keep in contact." Others enthusiastically agreed: "This is exactly what I was going to say! Every time she takes the time to send me a quick pic . . . there's nothing material that can match it!" Many women listed nonmaterial gifts: "My first IPs cherish me and my family and include us with updates and welcome us into their home quite frequently. That means more to me than any material item they could've gotten me. Even if it's a quick note to tell me something funny that the babies did, it means WAY more to me than anything."

Surrogates often discuss what gift to give at the first meeting with intended parents, what to get as a transfer gift, what gift to give when pregnancy is confirmed, and what to get for the baby shower. They write about how much they love to give gifts, but this is not the only, maybe not even the main, reason behind their gift practices. Repeated discussions reveal surrogates' eagerness to define the relationship with IPs as a personal one right from the beginning, and what better way to do this than with gifts? Yet, as a result of SMO stories, women are increasingly aware that bringing a gift may turn out to be a mistake; when IPs are visibly caught by surprise the surrogate may feel "silly."

Some occasions and some gifts cause more headaches than others. Countless discussions attest to the careful weighing of the pros and cons of giving; especially in the beginning of the journey it may be prudent to either refrain from gifting or select small and less personal gifts. Gifts at the beginning stages of surrogacy are more risky, and women are generally more careful not to give too soon, although many expressed caution only after they had given gifts. Early gifts can be problematic because they may celebrate a new relationship and a new identity before the fact. For example, when Mother's Day is too early in the journey a gift may be more disappointing than joyful. Surrogates deem it wiser to wait for confirmation of pregnancy or even until the end of the first trimester before giving motherhood-type gifts. SMO-ers articulate a similar reason for not giving at transfer: "if it ends up being a failed transfer I don't want her to look at the gift and have it be a reminder of a failed transfer."

Another common reason for caution before the parties had established patterns of giving and reciprocating is expressed in the following post: "I only got one gift for one of my potential IMs. It was a horseshoe charm on a chain. She did not get me anything and it was an awkward exchange. She opened it and put it away. She barely said thanks and that was the end of it. So I vote no gifts at transfer." SMO advice saved many women from feeling uncomfortable: "I took all your advice and didn't get anything and glad I didn't as they didn't bring a gift ([I] didn't expect one) but it would have been awkward." Feeling awkward and embarrassed is the result of misjudging the situation or misreading the relationship. Goffman pointed out that "Embarrassment has to do with unfulfilled expectations".[47] It is surrogates' expectation of being "on the same page" with their IPs, equally enthusiastic about the upcoming journey, that go unfulfilled in these situations. Surrogates are less constrained when their IPs gave a gift first: "My IM bought my daughter a birthday gift on only our second meeting ☺ So I wouldn't feel silly getting her a little something." In such instances, surrogates find giving gifts unproblematic because they are more confident that they and their IPs see the relationship the same way.

An intended mother admitted to getting her cues from SMO discussions, realizing how many surrogates give transfer day gifts: "I have given a transfer gift, though I probably wouldn't have unless I had heard about it on SMO." Surrogates, who find it hard not to give but are uncertain about what is appropriate to give, find "fertility bracelets," journals to record the journey, and other gifts that symbolize hope to be suitable choices. Especially creative surrogates symbolize fertility hopes in more playful ways; by giving and sending yellow and green ("fertility colors") flowers, balloons, and jelly beans.

Surrogates frequently discuss presents for other occasions as well. The more advanced the journey and the closer the relationship, the more personal the gifts. Gifts symbolically represent both the relationship between the surrogate and her couple and the IPs' changing status from intentions to parenthood. In the beginning, surrogates give and send flowers, local goodies, and other small gifts. Later in the journey they give or send picture frames, books on fetal development, ultrasound images, and the fetus' tape-recorded heartbeat. Lorraine, for example, gave this last gift: "at my last gyn appointment I heard the heart beat and taped it for IPs. They had no idea but I sent it to IM for Mothers' day."[48]

Closer to the birth surrogates send or give baby clothes, blankets, toys, and other baby items as well as scrapbooks or videotaped records of the journey. They also give intangible gifts; they provide detailed accounts of appointments when IPs cannot attend, take IPs' concerns seriously and forgo certain foods, drinks, and activities, and play IPs' voice-recorded stories to the fetus. There were some discussions about whether it was safe to put headphones directly on one's belly and how to avoid intruding on the privacy of these voice-recorded times of intimacy between IPs and their fetus-babies.[49]

Intentions and the problem of giving

Countless discussions notwithstanding, some questions and anxieties about gifts remain. Giving can become problematic when surrogates sense a lack of enthusiasm for their gifts or when IPs do not acknowledge or reciprocate them. Should these nonreciprocations be considered as indications that the surrogate has misread the clues or crossed a line or that IPs misunderstood her intentions? As much as they love to give gifts, a lot of surrogates worry about inappropriate timing and misread intentions. "Is a quilt too personal? I'm a HUGE quilter and wanted to throw together a little lap one or something and then a real cute one when we actually have the baby. Is that too personal or do you think it's ok if I have a close relationship with my IPs?"

If surrogates who have a close relationship worry about giving gifts, women whose IPs are standoffish worry even more:

still no news from my IPs. I called them last a few days before Christmas (when I had my level 2 U/S), to let them know about carrying a boy and a girl. IM sounded like she wanted to make amends, . . . [we] received a Christmas gift from them even. Since then, I have snail mailed tummy photos and pregnancy updates, and tried emailing them. . . . They have not attempted to call, email, or write in all that time. . . . I cannot understand them not wanting to keep in touch at least for the sake of appearances. I am dying to send them another gift (a diaper cake), just because I want to . . . part of the fun of surrogacy for me is spoiling the parents-to-be, but I feel like I am trying to buy their affection now, when I really just want the babies to have the best, and for their parents to feel connected in some way to their unborn children through me.

Surrogates often articulate the difference between giving as part of a relationship and giving because one wants to get something in return, whether it is compliance, attention, or affection. When the relationship is problematic, surrogates may read IPs' gifts as restitution or bribe and worry that IPs see the surrogate's gifts as an attempt to buy affection. It is easy to suspect the other party of having ulterior motives: IPs may try to ensure the surrogate's compliance; the surrogate may want the IPs' attention.

Gifts to surrogate babies are fraught with additional difficulties. SMO-ers are eager to show that their interest in the baby is anything but maternal and their gifts are not an intrusion into the new family. The following is a good example of some of the persistent difficulties of knowing what is appropriate: "can I hear from IPs what your surrogates got you for your baby that you found lovely and non-invasive? Can you also tell me IPs if there was anything that you would have found annoying receiving from your surrogate (I understand that I might be well over-thinking this)?" SMO-ers often express a desire to send Christmas and birthday presents to the child. The general advice on SMO is that surrogates should ask IPs if they object to such gifts. In less than close relationships, surrogates hope that their gift intentions will be regarded the way gifts from family friends are: a nice and friendly gesture.

But this is not always the case. Leslie reported that her IFs were against her sending gifts to the child and she thought of savings bonds as an alternative. She asked others how they interpreted the answer she received from her IFs: "Hi Leslie, we are undecided about the gifts thing, although it is very sweet, generous of you to want to. Saving bonds seem harmless enough. I will bring it up with

J. again . . . and ask around. We will have to discuss this more after
we gather information and talk about it." The following was a fairly
typical response to Leslie's question:

> I for the life of me cannot understand why this would be such an
> issue for IPs. If you had a family friend, would you accept gifts from
> them? At Christmastime, Easter, etc. Birthdays?? When your kids
> have friends, they're going to give gifts. Why for the life of me, an
> IP thinks it's even slightly acceptable to say, no you're not allowed
> to send gifts?? I mean. This is the greatest gift you could have given
> them. . . . I would hope that a surrogate would be at least considered
> a family friend.

Later, Leslie was given the provisional green light to "send occasional presents" as long as they did not confuse the child, and she
was very happy to be allowed to do so.

SMO-ers are often perplexed at IPs' reluctance to accept present
and discuss what to send that is "not offensive." Kaila, like many
others, looked for advice or at least support:

> I know my FIM (hi A.) will most likely read this, be surprised and
> tell me how very stupid I am for feeling this way . . . BUT . . . that's
> OK. I can't help it.
>
> So after my surro son was born I wanted SOOOO much to send
> gifts and cards and little things but I haven't yet because I didn't want
> to "crowd in" on their new family. This was their time and I didn't
> want to interfere in any way. I didn't want them to feel like I was
> going to be in their life "too much". But now he is 6 months and I am
> feeling like it's OK now. I still don't want to overstep my boundar-
> ies . . . but I would love to be able now to show them how much I do
> think of them and am so grateful they are part of our lives now. My
> girls speak of them so often. . . . It was so hard not to send anything
> for Xmas. So . . . anyone else ever feel this way? Do you send gifts,
> and are they welcomed?

Responses affirmed that surrogates do "feel this way": "I get
exactly what you mean. I think by now they'll be settled in (and
hopefully getting some more sleep) and thoughtful gifts are appropriate for special occasions." As Kaila thought, her intended mother
was reading the post: "You can send him anything you want to. . . .
I don't think it's intrusive! I told you when we started this journey I
wasn't looking for a business partner I was looking for an extension
of family and that's exactly what you (and your family) are to all
of us!"

As much as this is the reaction surrogates all hope—and are grateful—for, not everyone is this fortunate. Some women never even have their presents acknowledged: "I've always sent my surro 'babes' gifts for their birthdays and for Christmas. I sure hope they are appreciated."

One response illuminates a more complex and much less discussed aspect of gifts to one's surrobaby: "I can't imagine not buying her gifts . . . even though I'm not really on speaking terms with her mother anymore—it's still my way of letting the FAMILY know that I am thinking of them and wish them well." When IPs do not keep in contact with the surrogate, gifts to the baby can serve as a bridge to the parents. The baby cannot be expected to reciprocate; it is the IPs that would have to thank the giver. Surrogates sometimes send gifts to the child as a way to keep their tie to the family, although it is hard to acknowledge this without appearing manipulative. In some cases, however, women articulate their expectation of inviting some response:

> To try and entice a response, I sent a package out at the beginning
> of this week that I was told would arrive by today. . . . I spent a lot of
> time choosing the perfect gifts for the babies. . . . I know it's possible
> that the gift might not arrive on time, so I am not too worried about
> it. But I am still disappointed they haven't made any attempt to make
> contact. It's so sad.

Sending unrequited presents is a risky move for surrogates for a number of reasons. The couple may not acknowledge the gift, which is bad enough, but it is worse when they send it back or ask the surrogate not to send gifts ever again. Surrogates write about the embarrassment and humiliation they experience when couples do this, occasionally through a lawyer. Sometimes the surrogate's family expresses bafflement at her persistence, and she feels even more alone. When IPs do not acknowledge the gift, the surrogate often spend weeks wondering if they ever received it. When presents are returned, the surrogate feels devastated. Surrogates understand that refusing the gift is refusing to have a relationship: "It seems like the reason IPs may not want surrogates to give gifts is so there is no bond." Then adding insult to injury, when a surrogate insists on sending presents that are not welcome, fellow surrogates are not always sympathetic, sometimes accusing her of being manipulative and attention seeking.

The gift of trust

Almost as often as they debate on what to give and when to give, SMO-ers discuss gifts they receive from IPs. The theme of trust recurs in these discussions. Trust represents the appreciation surrogates value above all else: "I've never expected or wanted gifts—for me a trusting relationship is a treasure." Simply put, "I'm glad it's me they chose to carry their baby for them." Surrogates see trust as the return gift for their willingness to carry "the IPs' pregnancy." Some women think of IPs' trust as an even bigger gift and contend that it is IPs who give the most and surrogates should be the most grateful:

> They trusted ME to carry those precious little children, they trusted ME to grow them and get them here, you know what an honor that is??! I am incredibly thankful each and every day that these parents continue to let me be a part of these children's lives. Every visit, every hug, every kiss, every smile, seeing these parents, be, well, parents . . . how does the commercial go . . . priceless. We haven't and don't give near as much as you IPs have to give (and lose), we are honored to be trusted by you. You expand our hearts and our lives with what you entrust to us.

Many surrogates maintain that they are at least as lucky, if not more so, to have nice, appreciative, and trusting couples as IPs are to have good surrogates.

If surrogates understand carrying "precious little children" for others as a special honor and the delegating of pregnancy as an act of ultimate trust, it is not surprising that they feel privileged. Being the one who is trusted with the couple's baby and rewarded with the couples' time and attention bestows value on the surrogate. Myrna articulated this sentiment:

> after 8 years and countless couples, I finally have had the surrogacy experience with this last one that I dreamed of having for years prior to my ever becoming a surrogate. My IM and I are closer than sisters and I just love her to pieces. She and IF have given me more than I could have dreamed of, their gratitude, respect, trust and friendship.

As some women explain, they are reluctant to post too much about these gifts of trust and care, fearing to hurt the feelings of others who are treated less well. Yet they also want to educate potential and actual IPs on SMO about the importance of trust and appreciation:

Both sets [IPs] offered continuous support during my pregnancies. Both IMs attended EVERY doctor appointment which was much more important to me than any gift I could have received. I did get an occasional "we're thinking of you" gift along the way. Nothing huge, but flowers once when I was feeling particularly crappy, a few cards, a prenatal massage, phone calls, several lunches and simple gifts. Both IMs called at least once or twice a week to check on me and their children. One of the best things I got was a simple card sent out of the blue that said, "I don't believe in luck, but I believe in you." I can't say that I've seen many surrogates who expect the "royal" treatment. All of the ones I know just expect to be treated with the respect that every human being deserves. . . . There are times I have almost refrained from posting about the small, thoughtful gifts that my IPs have given me due to the fact that I know there are others out there that are just as deserving who aren't receiving anything more than their comp. . . . but at the same time I want potential IPs to understand that it doesn't take big or expensive items to make a surrogate feel appreciated. A simple card was enough to make me shed a few happy tears!

Surrogates love intangible gifts because they are understood as true signs of friendship and appreciation, free of the suspicions that sometimes accompany material gifts, namely, that they are meant to ensure surrogates' compliance and buy her goodwill. They love all the gifts they receive from their IPs when they see them as tokens of gratitude.

In one of the long threads about gifts, several surrogates reported being "spoiled" by their IPs. Elaine was one of them: "I was very spoiled through my pregnancy as were my kids. . . . I got 3 sets of diamonds through the whole pregnancy." Some others indirectly took up the issue of such gifts. "I doubt I will get the lavish gifts others have but I did not go into this to get gifts and presents. I choose a low fee so I could help a 'not-rich' family." The following is a typical reiteration of the importance of respect as the best gift: "nothing beats respecting, appreciating and caring for the person carrying your child and not treating her like a 'thing' but as some-one who also has emotional needs that should be respected. That can't be bought." Elaine came back to explain:

> I . . . posted about receiving diamonds. . . . I guess I should have said more than that I just received them. My FIM was my BEST friend. We talked every day 3–4 times . . . and [she] came up every weekend she could. That is all I ever wanted. I never expected the

gifts that I received and was mad at my IM and her mother for buying them. I was always treated with the upmost respect as was my entire family. When we found out we were pregnant with 3, everything changed. It was a more delicate situation and my FIPs stepped up the plate and went WAY over and beyond the call of duty. When my baby-sitter bailed on us, she went from full time to part time to spend 4 days a week with me while her Mom also went from full to part time to spend 2 days a week with us. My FIM quit her job and moved up here the very day I was put on hospital bedrest. No thinking involved. She raised my kids 24 hours a day. She did my laundry, cooked breakfast, lunch and dinner. Did the grocery shopping, and made sure my kids were happy which they were. I did not want them to suffer or have the pregnancy take a toll on them and it didn't because of her. That to me meant more than any gift, flowers, or phone call I could have gotten. She did everything in her power to make sure I was comfortable and not in pain. . . . she went above and beyond what our contract said or what I ever dreamed of. I LOVE her to this day for everything she did for my family.

In this light, the diamonds were gifts of love and expressions of appreciation. Elaine considered her former intended mother's concern, help, and friendship and the reciprocity they represented to be the most meaningful gifts.

The significance of intangible gifts is not lost on surrogates; material gifts may be too much like commodities people can buy for themselves:

Gifts to me are nothing, they come and go and I can buy myself "things" if I want them. I was spoiled in that my IM called me as often as she could. . . . I got thoughtful cards, and heartfelt emails and I KNEW their heart was with me all the time. When they were here I got hugs and my hand held, support, she cooked and cleaned my house, watched my boys and took care of me. . . . my most treasured moments were her and I sitting out on my front porch swing in our pajamas doing nothing.

For me though, this really is about the IMPORTANT things in life . . . my IPs treat me with the utmost respect, kindness, concern and love . . . it's no different than how my family and very close friends treat me . . . and THAT is exactly what I was looking for in a second surrogacy journey! When it comes to actual gift giving . . . the part that matters to me is the fact that my IPs actually *think* about it. . . . they pay attention to the little details in our lives . . . what we like, what we would appreciate most.

Many other women were equally thrilled when they received "thoughtful gifts," that is, gifts that attested to IPs' familiarity with the surrogate's preferences. In these instances surrogates see the intangible gifts of attention, consideration, and care embodied in the material gift, making the gift, no matter how small or trivial, unique and precious.

When one IM asked if she would be expected to buy her surrogate gifts, no one was offended by the question; replies pointed out that surrogates want friendship more than anything else. Surrogates sometimes contrast material presents with intangible gifts—trust, attention, time, and various manifestations of care and friendship—as if the latter were "more than" or the opposite of gifts: "It's more than the gifts. It's the phone calls and emails. Just the connection that makes you feel special and cared about." "I've never been given really lavish gifts. I've always been given thoughtful things that she knew would mean the world to me." SMO-ers denounce gifts when they resemble commodities that money can buy but embrace material as well as immaterial gifts when they stand for a relationship of respect and appreciation:

> It wasn't about how much money was spent and that's what I hear others saying as well. . . . It's just nice to be remembered and let's face it, everyone likes to feel appreciated. . . . I don't think that any of us . . . feel like our IPs "owe" us everything and have to repay us in gifts. . . . It was the emails and phone calls from my FIM . . . about everyday life and non-surro related stuff that made me feel like a friend, when they asked for advice or my thoughts on things . . . When my IPs email and ask how DH and the kids are, how they're doing in school, if they remember and ask if the child that was sick yesterday is feeling better etc.

As wives and mothers, surrogates want to have not just their own but also their family's sacrifices recognized and are delighted when IPs show concern for the whole family. As I argued before, surrogacy is ideally a relationship between two families, and this is clearly reflected in the high value surrogates place on IPs' gifts to the family. In a discussion on the "Parents via Surrogacy" forum about how to prepare and what to take to the delivery, an IM listed many items, adding that she was meaning to bring gifts to her surrogate's children but forgot. A gay intended father was more sensitive to the symbolism of such gifts:

> I also highly recommend gifts for your surrogate's child or children. When I showed up at the hospital, my surrogate's son was there help-

ing take care of the baby (she delivered before we had a chance to get there). When I gave him his gift he was so surprised and delighted and it meant a lot to his mom. I highly recommend it since the kids make a big sacrifice during the pregnancy.

Gift and money

If thoughtful gifts and gifts of thoughts are at one end of the spectrum, money gifts are at the other. Cash can be problematic because it looks too much like payment; posts about money gifts initiate serious discussions on SMO.

> My question is, how do I approach my IM about sending/giving me unnecessary cash? My fee is more than fair. The first time it happened was when I flew out to have my psych evaluation and medical screening. IM handed me some cash right before we parted ways. I told her it was not necessary, but she explained it as money to cover incidental travel expenses, food, whatever. I accepted the money but later I realized she gave me $200, which is way more than I needed. . . . IM sent us a lovely package in the mail with some things from their garden, a book for my daughter, etc. Although not necessary it was very sweet and I know they are trying to show their appreciation . . . am wonderfully blessed to have such a great situation with them. Anyway, in the package was a card with $300 cash in it . . . for no identified reason. . . . What do I do? . . . What would you do?

In this passage, the surrogate clearly differentiated between the items in the package that were presents and the cash that she was unsure about. Several women suggested putting the cash into a separate savings account and considering it an advance: "You can let your escrow know you were advanced x amount of money and to leave that much out of [the next] payment they send you." Some thought she could gift it back to the IPs after the birth or open a college saving account for the surrogate baby. But quite a few women were sensitive to the possibility of offending the intended parents since the money was meant as a gift: "accept it and say thank you." "It's obviously something that makes them feel good to do. It would probably hurt them to turn it down. If it makes you feel better, turn around and do something nice for them. Then look at what a nicer world you are all living in because of how thoughtful everyone is being." With the right intentions and the right way of giving, cash can be a gift and give rise to further gifts, weaving ties of reciprocal giving.

Money, however, can have unpleasant and cold connotations and some women had bad memories of such "gifts": "Sounds like my fIM . . . but to be quite frank, my IM used it as 'hush money.'

Money instead of communication. She couldn't email or call me, but she sure could mail a check! It made me very uncomfortable too." All the responses interpreted the money gift in the context of the relationship—mostly focusing on the rapport and the IPs' intentions as far as surrogates were able to assess. Money is more readily accepted and welcomed as a gift when the cash is intended to pay for things that make the surrogate's life easier during the pregnancy. Especially appreciated are payments for expenses that are not contractually covered. "My IPs paid for a house keeper to come every other week even though I wasn't on bed rest and I considered that a gift," wrote a surrogate in the last stages of a twin pregnancy that made it hard for her to move. Contracts very often specify IPs' obligation to pay for housekeeping help and/or childcare when bedrest is necessary. If they pay out of compassion when they are not obligated, most surrogates consider it a gift :

> My FIM used to give me cash near the end of my triplet pregnancy (here and there) to get the house cleaned weekly (instead of bi-monthly) or to have someone help with the laundry or to have the family go out to dinner so I didn't have to cook. . . . I gratefully accepted it. I very much appreciated it as I was having a hard time moving around. Even though I wasn't put on bed rest, my FIM knew that cooking, laundry, climbing stairs, and cleaning was getting very difficult for me. She also knew it was getting hard on my family picking up my slack. . . . But to accept cash prior to even transferring or becoming pregnant, I don't think I could accept it either.

Money is more acceptable as a gift when it is given on certain occasions and assigned for a specific purpose, as the above examples show, or is personalized in some other way, as in the following case:

> My IFs are extremely generous. . . . It would hurt their feelings if I gave it back to them. After H was born, they gave everyone in our family (dh and kids and me) a check and a letter stating how they felt about each one of us. It was very generous and very sweet. It would have crushed them if we didn't accept it.

Cash, which otherwise looks too much like payment, is considered a gift when the IPs have caring intentions that are tailored to the surrogate's needs and when they give in personalized ways. Personalized ways of giving or giving for specific purposes reveal knowledge of and familiarity with the surrogate and her family and are testimonies of IPs' concern, which, to surrogates, signify a personal relationship.

"Surrogacy requires an incredible sacrifice"

The gift of commitment

Surrogates frequently point out that personal relationships require sacrifice. Countless discussions attempt to define the range of hardships and risks that surrogates just have to accept. For example, when a newbie complained about a smallish procedure that had to be repeated, several women took up what they saw as the underlying issue:

> Wow I hope your IPs don't inconvenience you with anything that you feel is unnecessary. Blindsided with an additional uncomfortable and inconvenient procedure? . . .You do realize this is a surrogacy, right? Inconvenient things happen. Uncomfortable things happen. . . . Are you sure you have researched this? . . . I don't get what the problem is. . . . You do realize that this couple is probably spending thousands of dollars on this to become parents. The clinic is acting in THEIR best interest, so they can have a family. I just hope you have told this couple about how you feel "blindsided" and "inconvenienced" by this clinics protocol.

One surrogate highlighted her financial sacrifice: "I didn't get one dime from my IPs until I was pregnant. No testing fees, mileage, daycare, etc. There was a $500 transfer fee, which I waived. . . . I was perfectly happy with that arrangement." Annie, whose IM also occasionally posted on SMO, offered her opinion, thus sending a subtle message to her IM:

> We all have to go through this process and go into it expecting to jump through several hoops. . . . I am happy to do what I need to do in order to pass the screening process. I am sure the IPs would go above and beyond to do the same if they were in my position. I am doing this journey with my heart and not based on greed.

An intended mother chimed in, responding to the newbie's post: "Wow, reading this gives me the chills. . . . I could not imagine our surrogate being so cold and callous! I was happy to hear the other surrogates' responses!" No SMO-er wants to be "cold and callous," and as the above passages show, they often highlight the small sacrifices they made for their couples, frequently calling them necessary steps toward a successful surrogacy rather than sacrifice. Newbies often ask for advice about what responsibilities they should assume:

> This is my first time as a GS so I'm not sure what to expect, but I'm starting to get slightly annoyed. . . . I've been calling insurance

agencies, my OB and my hospital to get quotes for insurance rates
and out of pocket rates to compare prices. I'm happy to help, but I'm
feeling like some of this is not my responsibility and/or something
that should have been . . . looked into before now. Am I right or am
i being a baby? I have 3 kids, i work part time, I'm PTA secretary
and am now a girls scout leader and frankly, i don't have time to be
making 100 phone calls and emails a day.

Several surrogates took this opportunity to lecture the newbie
and others on SMO who may not be sufficiently willing to sacrifice:
"Surrogacy takes a lot of commitment and dedication. I have spent
countless hours, literally, on the phone, in waiting/exam rooms,
etc. to make a baby for my IFs." And even more bluntly: "this is
a part of surrogacy. . . . If you cannot commit to a few minutes
now how will you be able to make time later????" Amy's response
was a not-too-subtle statement about character: "Surrogacy is about
sacrifice . . . my life will come second to this pregnancy. I work
full-time, full-time student, mother of 3, so it can be done you just
have to be dedicated."

The limits of giving

These avowals of dedication and willingness to sacrifice notwithstanding, women also frequently debate the extent to which they
should or should not go to accommodate their IPs. They advocate
sacrifice but also collectively examine its limits. In a thread about
lessons learned, Nicky wrote the following:

> IPs are committed to having their baby, surros . . . commit to helping
> their IPs in this. To me it was a big thing. I committed myself to my
> IPs and have 2 successful journeys behind me. Regrets? Yes and No~
> maybe had I realized that red flags are important and to not brush
> them off because of a commitment. Then again I can't regret the lives
> that are here because of that commitment . . . but the commitment is
> to my family 1st and I have noticed that sometimes surrogacy can get
> so involved for a surro that she forgets what really matters. I've been
> there, in that tunnel vision. Hurting because of the commitment I
> made and realizing I was nothing more than a uterus. Because really
> isn't the commitment for the baby? Are surrogates a means to an
> end? . . . Surrogacy is a beautiful thing, even when it's painful, even
> when it hurts.

Fellow surrogates comforted Nicky, assuring her that creating
life was indeed worth the sacrifice. But responses also pointed
out the necessity of a more balanced giving. An IM, active on the

boards and admired for her views, offered her opinion about mutual commitment:

> It needs to be a healthy commitment, though. . . . IPs need to be as committed to being honorable to the surrogate as they are committed to pursuing having a family, and the surrogate needs to be at least as committed to their own family and needs as to those of the IPs. Are surrogates a means to an end? If you reduce it down, yes. IPs come to surrogacy because they lack the means. But if they value, even cherish, the possibility that is open to them because a surrogate is committed, it can be a wonderful and unique bonding shared experience. And I am saddened that your commitment was not met equally. That's an injustice.

Others focused on the "incorrigible proposition" about IPs' gratitude:

> SMs are a means to an end at the most basic level but that doesn't mean the whole experience can't be wonderful and joyous. . . . Even the IPs who I know had horrible relationships with their FSMs [former surrogate mothers] are still thankful . . . for the gift(s) that they received. Gifts that would not have been possible without YOU.

An intended mother reassured Nicky in the same vein:

> I am an IM. . . . There is not a day that goes by when i don't think about how amazing she [the surrogate] is. . . . i really want to believe in my heart that your FIPs think about the gift you have given them is the most amazing gift in the world and they know that you were their angel!! . . . i have to believe that every morning they wake up and realize what a blessing they have because of you!!!

Generally, surrogates remind one another that their own family is at least as important as the IPs'. However, there are a few exceptions, as the following case shows. In a sympathetic and supportive thread, fellow surrogates worried about Juliette, whose second journey with her international intended fathers ended in miscarriage and whose IFs were rumored to have "moved on without her." Juliette confirmed the rumor:

> Yes, it's true. A week ago, before my IF talked to our RE again, they were talking about coming here for an insemination and leaving Princess T (their daughter [Juliette's TS baby]) with me so that they could make a vacation out of it. Now, they've decided to move on without me. . . . I can't stop crying. Thank you so much for your support. It means so much. No one else understands. . . . This is part

of the email I sent to one of my IFs. I couldn't sleep and had to get my thoughts out of my head. . . . Today, I have to accept the fact that the moments with D and . . . . that I lost, every day spent riding to Connecticut, all my nausea, every pill, all the injections and bruises, the bloodwork and tests, every time I rested my foot in a stirrup, every class I missed taking, was all a waste of time, energy and pain. I won't be the one to tell you such good news. I won't be there to see your face when you are handed your child. . . . Instead, I will be 5,000 miles away. Insignificant. Irrelevant. Just "J," the "egg donor" and nothing more, ever.

A long time ago, D (my DH) warned me that I care too much. On the radio today, one of my favorites came on. '. . . Too long. Too late. Who was I to make you wait? Just one chance, just one breath—just in case there's just one left. Because you know I love you. I have loved you all along. And I miss you.'

This striking confessional post was received with unmitigated sympathy: "Wow Juliette, I'm in tears and I can feel your pain through your words. I'm so very very heartbroken for you and I think the IFs are making a big mistake." No one, other than Juliette's husband, pointed out that she "cared too much." Possibly, fellow surrogates saw that Juliette was in too much pain to be able to consider that she might have.

Nevertheless, in most "Lessons Learned" threads, women talk about both expectations that may have been too high and also sacrifices that in hindsight were excessive or misguided, as Ella's story exemplifies:

I came very close to death, thanks to the poorly done epidural before the emergency C section and then almost bled out, and my ^*(&#+)* FIPs never bothered to call me once they left the hospital with their baby.

Mind you, there were red flags throughout, but I disregarded them, babied my FIPs, put up with all sorts of business that NO surro should put up with, (the constant unrelenting nagging, the arrogant emails about the temperature of my bathwater, etc.). . . . I never ONCE thought about telling them back off or take it easy with the nagging, never once! Once I told FIM I was baking a cake. She asked me if her baby would be too hot being near the oven! CAN YOU BELIEVE IT? At the time I laughed but this is the type of stuff I dealt with! Questions are one thing—but this is downright hysterical BS!

They turned out to be the worst sort of cold blooded, heartless, cruel, misguided people, I have ever met. They acted afterwards like the baby was born early due to some fault of mine, (Oh did I mention they missed the delivery because, they said they HAD TO WORK) yes, they had to work! My nurse almost threw up when she heard this! . . . So they missed the near-dying episode and the delivery.

Never called me after they left the hospital! . . . Not one word of HOW ARE YOU?

My findings indicate that it is very difficult to know where being a "great surro" ends and sacrificing "too much" begins. In the final analysis, it is impossible to easily draw the line between "amazing journeys" and unwise sacrifices because surrogacy and pregnancy involve and sometimes necessitate giving in ways that no one intended or could have fully prepared for. One of the most common such situation is bed rest or hospitalization, sometimes for extended periods of time, mostly with multifetal pregnancy. Being unable to care for her children does hurt the surrogate and her family, yet by the time bedrest or hospitalization is necessary, there is no other course of action she can take. But even more to the point, these actions appear in a different light when the IPs are appreciative than when they are not. Yet IPs' appreciation and support is more likely to wane during difficult times. Couples are more stressed and anxious and may even suspect that the surrogate is somehow at fault.

In "amazing journeys" it is often the surrogate who is grateful for even the most ordinary manifestation of consideration, as the following story shows. Amy had "ups and downs" during her first GS but she and her husband "grew together" with the IPs. In the end, "everything was worth it":

But what I didn't know is the attachment I would feel for my couple. I never imagined in my wildest dreams that I would feel a loyalty to them that words cannot describe. I feel we are bonded as Souls meant to travel this World together to provide guidance and support and above all else a LOVE that families have. We are not bound by blood but LOVE which is way stronger!

Amy was ecstatic when her IPs agreed to do a sibling journey, and when the attempt failed she was grateful for her IPs' empathy for her:

We had a couple frozen embies left. . . . unfortunately that cycle failed. . . . [it was] harder for me than them. . . . I felt horrible. S. and K. comforted me even though it was just as big of a loss for them as it was [for] me. At that moment anytime they spoke with me they put my emotions before theirs. True friends! True Family!

As they tried again with the same egg donor, hoping that a cycle using fresh fertilized ova would be more successful than frozen ones, Amy's oldest son was hit by a pickup truck and was hospitalized "with a horrific head wound and broken leg." "Where did this leave our journey? S.'s words 'We can do frozen BE with your BOY honey—Do you need me I will be there tonight' After all the money they spent for a Fresh cycle it was the LAST thing she was thinking of! I love them every day for that! They are true family to me!"

Amy credits her couple for being true friends and highlights *their* sacrifice, and she does this again in her account of the birth when she needed an emergency C-section. She was asked to decide whether to undergo surgery right away or wait for a little longer until her husband, who was on his way, arrived. Being in pain and panicking, Amy was unable to make the decision and her IM asked the doctor to wait for the husband, which Amy recounts as a selfless act for which she is grateful.[50] "To my IPs THANK YOU for the LOVE you have given to me and my family." Amy's story is both similar to and different from Ella's—they both had accommodated their IPs and gone through hardships and emergency deliveries for them, but Amy was appreciated while Ella was not. The way the surrogacy ends provides a powerful lens for these two women, and surrogates in general, through which they see and evaluate their journeys.

Juliette's story of pain and Ella's bitter account also highlight surrogates' assumption that when their gift is not reciprocated and their sacrifice not appreciated fellow SMO-ers will listen and sympathize. Without expectations of support and understanding they may not post the narratives they did; stories of extreme, sometimes even unreasonable and often unrequited, giving would leave women too vulnerable to criticism. Who would risk her life and jeopardize her own family's financial and emotional well-being to provide strangers, who do not even appreciate her, with babies? These are some of the questions surrogates report hearing from family members, friends, and co-workers. The surrogate's motives, judgment, and intelligence may be questioned and insulted.

Sacrificing for people with whom she only imagined to be close or for relationships that have not been tested can be hazardous for a number of reasons: the surrogate may feel let down and used, she may also let down her own family in the process, and ultimately she may be criticized and discredited. On SMO, however, she may be reminded to put her family first or may be mocked for being "holier than thou," but in general, she is more likely to be criticized for being *unwilling* to "go above and beyond" than for going way beyond the call of duty.

Whether the journey goes well or not, SMO-ers enthusiastically advocate the position that surrogacy is a gift to all participants. Alyssa, whose IPs failed to keep in touch, echoed this sentiment when she commemorated the second anniversary of the birth:

> Everything became worth it with that cry that filled the room. . . . No one could take that moment from me. . . . Everyone says I gave this wonderful gift to someone that could not otherwise have it. I was given a gift as well, though. I was allowed to be involved in this journey in which I brought another human being into this world.

The surrogate is both a giver and a recipient. In this rendering of the journey, crystallized over the years, the surrogate rises above disappointments and gets the ultimate "boon" from fellow surrogates: the lasting distinction of having given the ultimate gift.[51] As Monica Konrad argued in her work on anonymous egg donors, "feeling special converts the gift into a vehicle of differentiation," turning the giver into a person of "presumed singularity."[52]

Notes

1. Melinda, e-mail communication, 22 April 2010.
2. Lorrain, e-mail communication, 18 May 2010.
3. Marilyn Strathern, "Partners and Consumers: Making Relations Visible," in *The Logic of the Gift: Toward an Ethic of Generosity,* ed. Alan D. Schrift (New York: Routledge, 1997), 301.
4. Elly Teman, *Birthing a Mother: The Surrogate Body and the Pregnant Self* (Berkeley: University of California Press, 2010), 209.
5. Heléna Ragoné, "The Gift of Life," in *Transformative Motherhood: On Giving and Getting in a Consumer Culture,* ed. Linda L. Layne (New York: New York University Press, 1999), 66.
6. Heléna Ragoné, *Surrogate Motherhood: Conceptions in the Heart* (Boulder, CO: Westview, 1994), 59.
7. Jonathan Parry, "The Gift, the Indian Gift, and the 'Indian Gift,'" *Man* 21, no. 3 (1986): 468.
8. Ibid.
9. Single embryo transfer (SET) has been increasingly advocated on SMO, but it is still very common to transfer two embryos, which can lead to multifetal pregnancy and higher risks.

10. In such situations surrogates who have a good relationship with IPs have an easier time choosing them to be present at the birth; husbands often have caretaking responsibilities at home anyway. When the relationship with IPs is strained, surrogates are more conflicted. Nevertheless, it appears that surrogates almost always think that IPs have a right to be at the birth even if they were not supportive of the surrogate during the pregnancy.

11. Surrogates offer this as a cost-saving measure or when the hospital does not provide a separate room for IPs. SMO-ers discuss the negatives, such as lack of privacy, but they also often report that the arrangement was gratifying because the intended mother was able to spend more time with the newborn and the surrogate enjoyed seeing, and helping, the new mother bond with the baby.

12. Teman found that Israeli surrogates think of "making another woman into a mother" as the most important and personalized gift they give (*Birthing a Mother*, 211).

13. Angelina, e-mail communication, 4 April 2006.

14. Marcel Mauss, *The Gift: The Form and Reason for Exchange in Archaic Societies* (New York: W.W. Norton, 1990). See also Strathern, "Partners and Consumers"; Monica Konrad, *Nameless Relations: Anonymity, Melanesia, and Reproductive Gift Exchange between British Ova Donors and Recipients* (New York: Berghahn, 2005); James Carrier, *Gifts and Commodities: Exchange and Western Capitalism Since 1700* (New York: Routledge, 1995).

15. James Carrier argued that Mauss's classic *The Gift* is valid and analytically useful to understand gift practices in modern capitalist societies. As opposed to commodities, which are exchanged in one-time transactions and payments end the relationship between the transacting parties, gifts establish obligations to receive and reciprocate. Carrier, *Gifts and Commodities*, 18–38.

16. Ibid., 21.

17. Ibid., 23.

18. Angelina, e-mail communication, 30 March 2006.

19. Teman, *Birthing a Mother*, 211

20. Georg Simmel, "Faithfulness and Gratitude," in *The Sociology of Georg Simmel*, ed. K.H. Wolff, 379–95 (New York: Free Press, 1950), 392.

21. Renée C. Fox and Judith P. Swazey, *The Courage to Fail. A Social View of Organ Transplants and Dialysis* (Chicago: University of Chicago Press, 1974), 333.

22. Ragoné argued that traditional surrogacy is a relationship of indebtedness; SMO-ers, however, do not use his word. Their use of "gratitude" is consistent with the understanding of surrogacy as a reciprocal but also voluntary relationship; debts and obligations beyond the contractually specified ones are not considered legitimate. Ragoné, "Gift of Life," 71.

23. Fred R. Berger, "Gratitude," *Ethics* 85, no. 4 (1975): 299.

24. Ibid., 299, 306.
25. Lorrain, e-mail communication, 30 May 2010.
26. Paul F. Camenisch, "Gift and Gratitude in Ethics," *Journal of Religious Ethics* 9, no. 1 (1981): 3.
27. Jonathan Parry and Maurice Bloch, eds., *Money and the Morality of Exchange* (New York: Cambridge University Press, 1989), 9; also Carrier, *Gifts and Commodities;* James Carrier, "Gifts, Commodities, and Social Relations: A Maussian View of Exchange," *Sociological Forum* 6, no. 1 (1991): 19–136.
28. Simmel, "Faithfulness and Gratitude," 392.
29. Berger, "Gift"; Camenish, "Gift and Gratitude."
30. Camenisch, "Gift and Gratitude," 19.
31. Berger, "Gratitude," 305.
32. Ava, e-mail communication, 2 May 2010.
33. As I noted in Chapter 2, it is ironic that surrogates bring up this possibility. Surrogates have no patience with suggestions that they cannot know how they will feel after birth.
34. It is worth noting that no one objected to calling surrogates "carriers," although in other discussions many surrogates dislike the term: "'Carrier' . . . how impersonal." "I've never cared for the term 'carrier,' . . . echoing other comments . . ., to me it sounds reminiscent of someone with a disease." However, surrogates often rally to defend this term when outsiders deride it, as Rush Limbaugh did. "Ha! Just emailed Rush Limbaugh about the proper terms for surrogacy . . . most people who are not involved in 'our' world have no idea. . . . I don't see anything wrong with . . . explaining why Keith Urban would refer to his surrogate as a gestational carrier."
35. Pollner explored the "ways in which assumptions are used as grounds for inference and action in concrete interactional settings." Mundane reasoning assumes an objective world, but only corrigible propositions give us information about the world, in that such propositions are admitted to be false if certain things happen in the world to discredit them. Incorrigible propositions, on the other hand, are compatible with any state of affairs and thus tell us nothing about the world. Presuppositions of various sorts limit the selection of explanations that account for the discrepancy between empirical reality and proposition. This is the case when surrogates propose that IPs are always grateful. Any behavior can be explained as "having a hard time dealing with or expressing their feelings," which leaves the assumption of gratitude intact, telling us nothing about the empirical reality. Melvin Pollner, "Mundane Reasoning," *Philosophy of the Social Sciences* 4, no. 1 (1974): 35–54.
36. Lee Taft, "Apology Subverted: The Commodification of Apology," *Yale Law Journal* 109, no. 5 (2000): 1137. Taft argues that in tort litigation, compensation does not satisfy the wronged parties who want

sincere apology. Admitting wrongdoing and showing remorse are moral actions that help the injured parties "heal," and surrogates also express this desire when they seek "closure" and "healing."

37. I documented some of the ways in which discussions were influenced and shaped by the tone of the initial post in Chapter 4 by quoting passages from three IMs' queries about money and surrogates' responses to them.

38. Sometimes SMO-ers go as far as saying that IPs have no choice but to look for a surrogate, while they can choose to be a surrogate or not.

39. Teman, *Birthing a Mother*, 253–55.

40. Carrier (*Gifts and Commodities*, 20) argues that the gift relationship is the social reproduction of people. In threads about arrangements for the delivery, surrogates correspond about trying to convince their couple to get a room in the hospital and be with the newborn. Surrogates are baffled by the IPs' preference not to, expecting them to "soak up all the time with their babies" after all the longing and waiting.

41. Linda's later posts have a new siggy showing that she had completed six traditional surrogacy journeys, but it is not clear if one of them was for this couple.

42. A few intended mothers confirmed these contentions, saying their husbands were "standoffish, uncomfortable, and weird" around insemination time and did everything to delay, and the IM had to "drag him kicking and screaming" even though they very much wanted to be fathers. Several IMs reported that things got better and more relaxed after the surrogate got pregnant. These and many other threads I read about inseminations contradict some feminists' claims about "patriarchal practices," whereby men coerce their wives to consent to such surrogacy arrangements. See, e.g., Christine Overall, *Ethics and Human Reproduction: A Feminist Analysis* (Boston: Allen and Unwin, 1987); Andrea Dworkin, *Right-Wing Women* (London: Women's Press, 1987).

43. Accounts of the gifts IPs give are consistent with the gift-related advice on the message boards, and the gifts are similar to gifts exchanged in many other social situations when the parties are not very close.

44. Teman, *Birthing a Mother*, 220.

45. Teman, *Birthing a Mother*, 212.

46. Many more threads discuss women's disappointment over not being invited to the baby shower, but nobody voiced unhappiness about not getting gifts.

47. Erving Goffman, "Embarrassment and Social Organization," *American Journal of Sociology* 62, no. 3 (1956): 268.

48. Lorraine, e-mail communication, 21 May 2010.

49. The most common suggestions were that the surrogate put in earplugs or earphones while playing the IPs' recording or put the player device on her belly and place a pillow on it.

50. It seems likely that the doctor would not have asked whether Amy wanted to wait if he had thought the baby was in immediate danger. It may be that the IM's decision was a considerate gesture for the woman who was undergoing emergency surgery for her, rather than a selfless sacrifice.
51. Just as Campbell's heroes, the surrogate shares her "boon" with the world. While the baby is not hers, her achievement and gain are tied to carrying and birthing a baby for others. Joseph Campbell, *The Hero with a Thousand Faces* (Novato, CA: New World Library, 2008).
52. Monica Konrad, *Nameless Relations*, 74.

CONCLUSION

Through frequent and ongoing communication, women have created an online world of advice and support and along the way negotiated surrogacy-related views, behaviors, and feelings. Over the years members have brought their stories to the message boards, and newcomers have absorbed an increasing and increasingly rich body of medical, legal, relational, and emotional knowledge. Oldtimers and newcomers have debated issues and settled on solutions, sometimes only to modify them later. Some questions recurred and persisted while others were answered definitively and disappeared from the boards.

Collectively, SMO-ers have worked out the ethos of surrogacy, settled questions about feelings and behaviors in a range of situations, and defined what it is to be "a great surro." They did not set out to do all this, but neither are the collective definitions of surrogacy-related ideas and behaviors simply a byproduct of communications associated with advice and support. Communication and definitions go hand in hand; they produce and reproduce one another. Drawing on the insight of symbolic interactionism, what is at stake for surrogates is both self-identity as helpful, giving people and group membership as being one of "the wonderful ladies" on SMO.

Throughout the book, I have argued that surrogates form and negotiate collective understandings of surrogacy-related events, behaviors, and feelings. In their quest to make sense of a reproductive practice that involves both their bodies and their sense of self, women draw from and combine cultural understandings about life, family, relatedness, intimacy, and reciprocity. SMO provides the "opportunity structure" for construction and negotiation of these meanings.[1] "While meanings are negotiated, they are never negotiated anew," Gary Fine emphasized, and this is what we see in discussions among surrogates.[2]

They draw from existing framings and imagery, formulated by agencies, surrogacy professionals, and other parties to surrogacy. They also draw from cultural understandings concerning family, children, and pregnancy. On the message boards we can catch a glimpse of the narrative construction of the online world of surrogacy. In this "semiotic community" women make "use of a semiotic code to do something in the world": to carry babies for others and make sense of this practice in the context of competing interpretations.[3] As Sewell argued, using the semiotic code means attaching "abstractly available symbols to concrete things or circumstances and thereby to posit something about them."[4]

Journey

The "journey" is a case in point; it signifies the shared goal-oriented and transformative path that came to symbolize the contractual arrangement between surrogates and intended parents. When SMO-ers remind one another "to honor the journey" they do not mean their individual arrangements, which may or may not have turned out well; rather, they urge one another to honor surrogacy as a social practice and to uphold its moral value. However, time and again women also insist that every journey is different, seemingly contradicting the conceptualization of surrogacy as a social practice. Even as they offer advice to others, surrogates often conclude with "it's just me," reiterate that "everyone is different," and that they "cannot speak for others." What we witness on SMO is the balancing of two collective definitions of surrogacy. On the one hand, surrogacy is understood as a unique relationship between unique people; on the other hand, it is a practice women can meaningfully shape together as it transcends individual arrangements.

Surrogates emphasize their love for, and unique relationship with, their couple and also discuss and debate the obligations, actions, and emotional reactions that follow from such a relationship, thus collectively formulating common ground. When IPs fail to keep their promise of continued contact, surrogates see it as a betrayal—rather than a breach of contract—which is consistent with the conceptualization of the journey as one of shared love. As I documented in previous chapters, SMO-ers work out ways to come to terms with less-than-happy developments together. Emphasis on the uniqueness of each journey notwithstanding, negotiating obligations, actions, and emotional responses involves a "collective effort to mold feeling."[5]

These collective negotiations can be contentious, but SMO discussions generally recognize and validate feelings of disappointment. Still, while these debates acknowledge sadness and anger, they tend to censure purely negative feelings about the journey and applaud efforts to overcome disappointments. This way, surrogates effectively advocate and endorse some alternative emotional stances, and thus alternative meanings for the journey, such as feelings of pride, even moral superiority. William Reddy contended that "communities systematically seek to train emotions, to idealize some, to condemn others."[6] The online surrogacy community is doing just this. Love of family and the preciousness of children is the common ground for surrogates and intended parents, but much cultural and emotional work is required to navigate surrogate journeys and to gain recognition in the SMO community.

Stories of sustained effort to find IPs to click with and love IPs one has matched with are always greeted with enthusiastic support on the boards. Being too dependent on IPs' love is not condoned, however. Just as women are supposed to take charge of their journey by doing research on the legal and medical aspects of surrogacy, they are responsible for managing their emotions and the emotional impact of their IPs' actions.

My findings indicate that emotion management is achieved through interactions with others and without institutional support. Emotional expression and control are part of the evolving negotiation of the standards of behavior SMO-ers are invested in, all the while claiming that standards do not apply to these individual journeys. A "great surrogate" is well informed, smart, responsible, reliable, helpful, compassionate, loving, and yet emotionally independent.

In formulating these standards, women draw on culturally feminine values, such as empathy and generosity, as well as on the culturally American values of autonomy, rationality, and self-control. It is hard to live up to these standards but there is much at stake, and the stakes are very similar for all surrogates. They may feel "ditched" and emotionally crushed when IPs do not stay in touch, or they may be able to be "the better person" and salvage their self-respect. They may gain authority, recognition, and admiration on SMO, or they may be chastised and criticized by other surrogates, the very people who are supposed to understand and support them. They may also collectively gain validation for their own life choices that prioritized children and family. The emotional monitoring and adjusting that surrogates engage in are tied to collective definitions of goals.

SMO offered a considerably larger forum for self-organized social control and collective definitions of worthiness[7] than agency-organized support groups did.[8] This online forum provided opportunities for information and guidance; it also facilitated not only the telling of stories but also their circulation that keeps these stories alive.

Geertz emphasized the importance of particular symbolic vehicles, such as stories, in the creation of collective definitions and a shared outlook.[9] I have explored how shared emotional experience, goals, and outlook are achieved through stories and discussions and the consequences it has for expectations for and assessments of the journey. Surrogates' online discussions, birth stories, and diaries are vehicles for meaning making. The message they most often carry is of a journey of ultimate meaning and purpose—a journey that is a test of character and validation of personal worth.

Ideally, the romance of surrogacy is lived in a "perfect match." However, the framework of love does not have to be threatened by lack of reciprocation from intended parents. By constructing and intensifying emotions of pride and also acknowledging pain, women work out new emotional reactions and courses of action: disappointments do not have to discredit the love or undercut the purpose as long as women "honor the journey." The "heart" symbolically stands not only for emotions and identity but also for strength and stability.[10]

SMO-ers readily share their stories of both joy and anguish because they believe that these stories instruct and comfort others. Women who had "perfect journeys" may hold back, afraid to upset others who had more disappointing experiences. However, women tend to remind everyone that journeys have some difficulties and emotional ups and downs. "I think we all here have our share of [pain]. . . . All we can do is honor the journey and try to move on and know that we did the BEST we could as surrogates." This emotional regime strengthens resolve; surrogates' collective emotional work has contributed to the enthusiasm to repeatedly bear children for others.

The "creative cultural actions" I documented in this book have enabled women to establish as well as retain the moral value and purpose of surrogacy.[11] Surrogates say that creating life, parents, and families is worth more than any payment. Upholding the sacredness of life most often involves contrasting it with monetary values; through these comparisons surrogates creatively work out the incommensurability of life. However, we have also seen that agreement about and timely payments of compensation represent not simply "well-deserved money" but also the care and appreciation surrogates wish to receive from their couple.

Surrogates navigate between two worlds in more ways than one. They both construct and challenge boundaries between the world of money and self-interest, on the one hand, and the world of love and altruism, on the other. They also move between a world in which they interact with IPs and various professionals in the field and the world of SMO, where they communicate with fellow surrogates. It is in these SMO communications that they collectively work out a "rule of conduct" that guides them in this new reproductive realm, in which obligations and expectations are neither clear-cut nor uniformly agreed upon.[12] Surrogates debate these rules, but once they come to some general agreement they espouse and defend them.

Goffman argued that when people become invested in rule maintenance, they also "become committed to a particular image of self."[13] I have documented how SMO-ers define and maintain the collective self-image of intelligent, giving, strong, and altruistic women. However, this self-image is not always reflected back at surrogates in the mirror of the IPs' treatment of them. Nevertheless, women on SMO are in a reasonably good position to remedy this. Both respect and disrespect from IPs function as currency that can be exchanged for respect on the message boards if the surrogate presents herself and her case in a balanced manner, with due deference to others' points of view.

Gift and Market

How can we think about the relationships and transactions of surrogacy in the context of the rich and creative meanings we see emerging on the message boards? Ostensibly, there is a tension between personal and contractual framings of surrogacy. Surrogates insist that all journeys are different, but there is standardization in quite a few areas, as we can surmise from these same narratives. By applauding and rewarding some behaviors and feelings, surrogates, albeit unintentionally, bring about standardization in the definition of the "good surrogate."

Lawyers have worked out increasingly long and progressively more standardized surrogacy contracts, and surrogates themselves have been pushing for more detailed and precise contractual specifications. Agencies offer standardized categories of compensation and contract and have devised routine ways to proceed. IPs and indy surrogates research agency websites and SMO message boards to find "going rates" and sample contracts. Surrogates talk about asking for "less than average," "average," or, much less frequently, "higher than average" fees, and despite reiterations of "only you know what you need" they discuss a growing list of "must have" contractual provisions.

Still, surrogacy is neither an occupation nor a profession, and surrogates are quite hostile to these designations.[14] SMO-ers say that everyone with "a working uterus" can be a surrogate, although they also maintain that it takes much more to be a good surrogate. A good surrogate needs to be smart, independent, altruistic, and willing to sacrifice. When they insist that they are "not in the profession," women often contrast surrogates with surrogacy professionals, such as doctors and lawyers. However, SMO-ers tend to embrace the notion that professional behavior, in the sense of being rational and reliable, is a good thing in surrogacy. Surrogacy is not an occupation either; surrogates cannot count on easily finding IPs to match with, nor can they take smooth pregnancies and even achieving pregnancy for granted, thus they cannot count on it for income. They do not make a living by carrying babies for others and carefully earmark the money they receive as compensation, as special money to be used for certain purposes only.

Nevertheless, Everett Hughes's distinction between license and mandate is well taken here.[15] Anyone who is cleared by medical professionals and finds IPs can be a surrogate. No special license is required, but SMO-ers have increasingly claimed "a mandate to define . . . proper conduct" as well as "modes of thinking and belief" for themselves and others.[16] Surrogates are not the only participants whose actions, verbal and otherwise, impact assisted reproduction; clinics, doctors, lawyers, and agency personnel are major players as well. But unlike doctors, lawyers, and agency and clinic staff, surrogates are not only nonprofessional but also noninstitutional actors; with the help of the Internet they self-organize and learn to navigate institutional settings in ways that leave room for creative relational work.

Nina Bandelj predicted that "relational work will be more prominent and elaborate in economic situations that are more uncertain and ambiguous" because these situations are more open-ended and "require more elaboration of the nature of the relationship."[17] Bandelj is right; women repeatedly and at length elaborate the nature of the relationship with intended parents precisely because surrogacy carries ambiguous meanings. SMO-ers reject meanings such as "baby selling," "reproductive service," and being an "employee" by rejecting the notion that money is for the baby or for gestational service. They embrace characterizations such as "two families helping each other"; thus it is possible to see money as the IPs' way of helping their surrogate.

Surrogacy thus has market and nonmarket characteristics and is being powerfully shaped by contradictory desires, practices, and interests; it is fashioned and refashioned by interactions.

Why is there so little empirical exploration of these rich interactions between monetary and other values and between the market logic and altruism? Viviana Zelizer's contention, articulated more than thirty years ago, is still very much to the point: "Perhaps the absorption of many social scientists with 'market' models and the notion of economic man led them and others to disregard certain complexities in the interaction between the market and human values."[18] Rene Almeling has recently summarized this same tendency: "Abstract distinctions between economy and society, between commodity and gift, are common in discussions of commodification, but empirical research in economic sociology challenges the idea of a stark dichotomy between market processes and social life."[19]

Empirical studies on surrogacy and egg, sperm, and organ donation have documented the tremendously rich, creative, and complex ways in which "people articulate the relationship between moral and economic classification in their personal interactions and activities."[20] Throughout the book I have documented the ways in which surrogates debate and negotiate the relationship between moral and economic actions and meanings. Zelizier hypothesized that sacralizing efforts increase in situations when "profanation of the sacred" occurs, as they did when life insurance became a lucrative business.

There is a powerful normative stigma associated with monetized practices when it comes to life (or death): "to save and to heal is holier than to sell."[21] As we have seen, SMO-ers vow not only to nurture life but also to heal the wounds of infertility by giving IPs the gift of life. The profanation they are consistently reminded of—even if not always accused of—by frequent and public questions and comments about how much they are paid is a mighty incentive for the sacralization of the life they help create.

Through sustained discussions they reconcile the cultural opposites of life and payment, and instead of money profaning life, it is the sacredness of life, which surrogates trace back to Petri dishes and

IPs' dreams of a baby, that surrogates emphasize. These "much loved and desired babies" are always described as precious life and IPs as "deserving"; in stark contrast to critics' fears of commodification of pregnancy and babies, we actually see ritualization of surrogates' "ultimate giving" and a heightened sacralization of life. Surrogacy is a new frontier in many ways and offers us new insights into the relational nature of human practices. Ethnographic explorations of these practices also help us add to the range of empirical answers about how gift and market exchange relate to moral worth.[22]

Surrogates champion empathy, altruism, and sacrifice as the morally right response to "deserving" people's quest to overcome infertility. Simultaneously, they uphold the moral value of both equality and reciprocity. SMO-ers believe that their willingness to help others should not undermine the basic equality of lives; as precious as they are, the babies they carry should not be valued more than the surrogate's own children, whose lives are impacted by the fact that their mother carries for others. Compensation for their labors and reimbursement for expenses are financial means to guarantee that surrogates and their families do not suffer undue hardships for helping others and their giving is reciprocated. Money, rather than undermining moral values, enables surrogates to uphold the ideals of equality and reciprocity.

Compensated (or as it is also called, "commercial") surrogacy is both a market concept and a moral one. Participants, most often strangers without any previous relationship, enter this contractual arrangement as a free choice; however, the babies surrogates carry and birth are not commodities but unique, inalienable, and non-fungible persons that surrogates and many IPs believe establish a lifelong bond between giver and recipient. Some people find this bond unsettling while others embrace it; with no social precedents to what such a relationships is and what it entails, the parties work out the rules of engagement of contractual intimacy.

In this book, I implicitly took up Margaret Radin's question: "Does the rightness or wrongness of any transaction where money changes hands, and also where parental rights change hands, depend in any way on how we think of it?"[23] I brought my data to bear on this question not because I wanted to answer the normative problem of right or wrong but because the ways in which surrogates collectively think about these questions do provide *them* with answers about the moral rightness of surrogacy.

Healy suggested that we think of gifts and market exchange not as opposites, "belonging to different social worlds," but as "tendencies that can be found together to greater or lesser degrees in the same society."[24] SMO-ers' discussions articulate the coexistence and interrelatedness of money and gift, contract and love. As with other new developments in market societies, it is organizational and cultural work to fashion, negotiate, and make sense of these tendencies of gift and market exchange and to work out their practical and moral implications.

Notes

1. Gary A. Fine, "The Sociology of the Local: Action and Its Publics," *Sociological Theory* 28, no. 4 (2010): 356.
2. Ibid. Sewell makes a similar point. William H. Sewell, Jr., "The Concept(s) of Culture," in *Beyond the Cultural Turn: New Directions in the Study of Society and Culture,* ed. V.E. Bonnell and L. Hunt (Berkeley: University of California Press, 1999).
3. Sewell, "Concept(s) of Culture," 51. Zelizer's study of life insurance explores a similar situation historically, capturing the changing meaning of the monetary evaluation of death in the nineteenth century and documents its implications for the business of insuring life. Viviana A. Zelizer, "Human Values and the Market: The Case of Life Insurance and Death in 19th-Century America," *American Journal of Sociology* 84, no. 3: 591–610.
4. Sewell, "Concept(s) of Culture," 51.
5. William M. Reddy, *The Navigation of Feeling. A Framework for the History of Emotions* (Cambridge: Cambridge University Press, 2001), 59.
6. Ibid., 324.
7. A commonly used term in the sociological literature is "self-empowerment"; however, I prefer to use a more descriptive term. Surrogates' discussions revolve around their own worthiness as surrogates and as people and around the value of giving, rather than power. In fact, "value," "worth," and "valuation" are frequently used terms on the message boards, while "power" is used extremely rarely.
8. Heléna Ragoné, *Surrogate Motherhood: Conceptions in the Heart* (Boulder, CO: Westview, 1994), 42–44.
9. Clifford Geertz, *Interpretation of Cultures* (New York: Basic Books, 1973).
10. Elly Teman, *Birthing a Mother: The Surrogate Body and the Pregnant Self* (Berkeley: University of California Press, 2010), 68.
11. Sewell, "Concept(s) of Culture," 51.
12. Erving Goffman, "The Nature of Deference and Demeanor," *American Anthropologist* 58, no. 3 (1956): 473.
13. Ibid., 474.

14. "The professionals claim the exclusive right to practice, as a vocation, the arts which they profess to know," wrote Everett Hughes. E.C. Hughes, *On Work, Race, and the Sociological Imagination* (Chicago: University of Chicago Press, 1994), 38.

15. Ibid., 25–26.

16. Ibid., 25.

17. Nina Bandelj, "Relational Work and Economic Sociology," *Politics and Society* 40, no. 2 (2012): 185.

18. Zelizer, "Human Values," 592.

19. Rene Almeling, "Gender and the Value of Bodily Goods: Commodification in Egg and Sperm Donation," *Law and Contemporary Problems* 72, no. 3 (2009): 38.

20. Marion Fourcade, "Theories of Markets and Theories of Society," *American Behavioral Scientist* 50, no. 8 (2007): 1028.

21. Zelizer, "Human Values," 607.

22. Marion Fourcade and Kieran Healy, "Moral Views of Market Society," *Annual Review of Sociology* 33 (2007): 301.

23. Margaret Jane Radin, "What, If Anything, Is Wrong with Baby Selling?" *Pacific Law Review* 26, no. 2 (1995): 136. Radin's answer to this question is yes, although she finds it surprising that the moral evaluation of the transaction depends to some extent on how we think about it.

24. Kieran Healy, *Last Best Gifts, Last Best Gifts: Altruism and the Market for Human Blood and Organs* (Chicago: University of Chicago Press, 2006), 16.

BIBLIOGRAPHY

Abbott, Andrew. "Of Time and Space: The Contemporary Relevance of the Chicago School." *Social Forces* 75, no. 4 (1997): 1149–82.

Abend, Gabriel. "The Meaning of 'Theory.'" *Sociological Theory* 26, no. 2 (2008): 173–99.

Addelson, Kathryn P. "The Emergence of the Fetus." In *Fetal Subjects, Feminist Positions,* edited by Lynn M. Morgan and Meredith W. Michaels, 26–42. Philadelphia: University of Pennsylvania Press, 1999.

Adler, Nancy E., Susan Keyes, and Patricia Robertson. "Psychological Issues in New Reproductive Technologies: Pregnancy-Inducing Technology and Diagnostic Screening." In *Women and New Reproductive Technologies: Medical, Psychological, Legal, and Ethical Dilemmas,* edited by Judith Rodin and Aila Collins. Hillsdale, NJ: Lawrence Erlbaum, 1991.

Allen, Charlotte. "Womb for Rent." *The Weekly Standard,* 7 October 2013, 29.

Almeling, Rene. "Gender and the Value of Bodily Goods: Commodification in Egg and Sperm Donation." *Law and Contemporary Problems* 72, no. 3 (2009): 37–58.

———. *Sex Cells: The Medical Market for Eggs and Sperm.* Berkeley: University of California Press, 2010.

Anderson, Elijah. *Code of the Street: Decency, Violence, and the Moral Life of the Inner City.* New York: W.W. Norton, 1999.

———. "The Ideologically Driven Critique." *American Journal of Sociology* 107, no. 6 (2002): 1533–50.

———. "Jelly's Place: An Ethnographic Memoir." *Symbolic Interaction* 26, no. 2 (2003): 217–37.

Anderson, Elizabeth S. "Is Women's Labor a Commodity?" *Philosophy and Public Affairs* 19, no. 1 (1990): 71–92.

Andrews, Lori. *New Conceptions.* New York: Ballantine, 1985.

Anleu, Sharyn R. "Surrogacy: For Love but Not for Money?" *Gender and Society* 6 (1992): 30–48.

Arrow, Kenneth J. "Invaluable Goods." *Journal of Economic Literature* 35, no. 2 (1997): 757–765.

Bahr, Howard and Kathleen S. Bahr. "Families and Self-Sacrifice: Alternative Models and Meanings for Family Theory." *Social Forces* 79, no. 4 (2001): 1231–58.

Bandelj, Nina. "Relational Work and Economic Sociology." *Politics and Society* 40, no. 2 (2012): 175–201.

Baumann, Gerd. "Ritual Implicates 'Others': Rereading Durkheim in a Plural Society." In *Understanding Rituals,* edited by Daniel de Coppet, 97–116. New York: Routledge, 1992.

Baer, Judith A. *Ironic Freedom: Personal Choice, Public Policy, and the Paradox of Reform.* New York: Palgrave Macmillan, 2013.

Becker, Gay. *The Elusive Embryo: How Women and Men Approach New Reproductive Technologies.* Berkeley: University of California Press, 2000.

Becker, Howard S. *Doing Things Together.* Evanston, IL: Northwestern University Press, 1986.

———. "The Epistemology of Qualitative Research." In *Ethnography and Human Development: Context and Meaning in Social Inquiry,* edited by Richard Jessor, Anne Colby, and Richard A. Shweder. Chicago: University of Chicago Press, 1996.

———. *Outsiders.* The Free Press, New York, NY, 1963

———. *Tricks of the Trade.* Chicago: University of Chicago Press, 1998.

———. *Sociological Work.* New Brunswick, NJ: Transaction Books, 1970.

Bellah, Robert, Richard Madsen, William M. Sullivan, Ann Swidler, and Steven M. Tipton. *Habits of the Heart: Individualism and Commitment in American Life.* Berkeley: University of California Press, 1985.

Bender, Courtney. *Heaven's Kitchen: Living Religion at God's Love We Deliver.* Chicago: University of Chicago Press, 2003.

Ben-Ze'ev, Aaron. *The Subtlety of Emotions.* Cambridge, MA: MIT Press, 2000.

Berend, Zsuzsa. "Surrogate Losses: Understandings of Pregnancy Loss and Assisted Reproduction among Surrogate Mothers," *Medical Anthropology Quarterly* 24, no. 2 (2010): 240–62.

———. "'We Are All Carrying Someone Else's Child!': Relatedness and Relationships in Third-Party Reproduction," *American Anthropologist* 118, no. 1 (2016):24-36.

Berger, Fred R. "Gratitude." *Ethics* 85, no. 4 (1975): 298–309.

Berkhout, Suze G. "Buns in the Oven: Objectification, Surrogacy, and Women's Autonomy." *Social Theory and Practice* 34, no. 1 (2008): 95–117.

Blumer, Herbert. *Symbolic Interactionism: Perspective and Method.* Englewood Cliffs, NJ: Prentice-Hall, 1969.

Boli, John. "The Economic Absorption of the Sacred." In *Rethinking Materialism: Perspectives on the Spiritual Dimension of Economic Behavior,* edited by Robert Wuthnow, 93–115. Grand Rapids, MI: Eerdmans, 1995.

Boulding, Kenneth. *The Economy of Love and Fear.* Belmont, CA: Wadsworth, 1973.

Bruckman, Amy. "Identity Workshop: Emergent Social and Psychological Phenomena in Text-Based Virtual Reality." Unpublished manuscript.

MIT Media Laboratory, 1992. http://www.academia.edu/2888780/ Identity_Workshop:

Bruner, Jerome. *Making Stories: Law, Literature, Life.* Cambridge, MA: Harvard University Press, 2003.

———. "The Narrative Construction of Reality." *Critical Inquiry* 18, no. 1 (1991): 1–21.

Camenish, Paul F. "Gift and Gratitude in Ethics." *Journal of Religious Ethics* 9, no. 1 (1981): 1–34.

Campbell, Joseph. *The Hero with a Thousand Faces.* Novato, CA: New World Library, 2008.

Camenisch, Paul F. "Gift and Gratitude in Ethics." *Journal of Religious Ethics* 9, no. 1 (1981): 1–34.

Carrier, James. *Gifts and Commodities: Exchange and Western Capitalism Since 1700.* New York: Routledge, 1995.

———. "Gifts, Commodities, and Social Relations: A Maussian View of Exchange." *Sociological Forum* 6, no. 1 (1991): 19–136.

Casper, Monica J. "Reframing and Grounding Nonhuman Agency: What Makes a Fetus an Agent?" *American Behavioral Scientist* 37, no. 6 (1994): 839–56.

Cavanagh, Allison. "Behavior in Public? Ethics in Online Ethnography." *Cybersociology Magazine: Research Methodology* 6 (1999). Accessed 28 November 2009. http://www.cybersociology.com/files/6_2_ethicsinonlineethnog.html.

Cerulo, Karen A. "Reframing Sociological Concepts for a Brave New (Virtual?) World." *Sociological Inquiry* 67, no. 1 (1997): 48–58.

Cerulo, Karen A., Janet M. Ruane, and Mary Chayko. "Technological Ties That Bind: Media-Generated Primary Groups." *Communication Research* 19, no. 1 (1992): 109–29.

Charmaz, Kathy. "Grounded Theory." In *Contemporary Field Research: Perspectives and Formulations.* 2nd ed. Edited by R.M. Emerson. Prospect Heights, IL: Waveland, 2001.

Chase, Susan E. and Mary F. Rogers. *Mothers and Children: Feminist Analyses and Personal Narratives.* New Brunswick, NJ: Rutgers University Press, 2001.

Clore, Gerald L. "For Love or Money: Some Emotional Foundations of Rationality." *Chicago-Kent Law Review* 80, no. 3 (2005): 1151–65.

Cohen, Anthony. *The Symbolic Construction of Community.* London: Tavistock, 1985.

Collier, Jane, Michelle Z. Rosaldo, and Sylvia Yanagisako. "Is There a Family? New Anthropological Views." In *Rethinking the Family*, edited by Barrie Thorne with Marilyn Yalom. New York: Longman, 1982.

Collier, Jane and Sylvia Yanagisako. "Toward a Unified Analysis of Gender and Kinship." In *Gender and Kinship: Essays toward a Unified Analysis*, 14–52. Stanford, CA: Stanford University Press, 1987.

Corbin, Juliette and Anselm Strauss. *Basics of Qualitative Research: Techniques and Procedures for Developing Grounded Theory.* 3rd ed. Los Angeles: Sage, 2008.

Corea, Gena. *The Mother Machine: Reproductive Technology from Artificial Insemination to Artificial Wombs.* New York: Harper & Row, 1985.

Correll, Shelley. "The Ethnography of an Electronic Bar: The Lesbian Café." *Journal of Contemporary Ethnography* 24, no. 3 (1995): 270–98.

Costigan, James T. "Introduction: Forests, Trees, and Internet Research." In *Doing Internet Research: Critical Issues and Methods for Examining the Net,* edited by Steven G. Jones. Thousand Oaks, CA: Sage, 1999.

Cussins, Charis. "Producing Reproduction: Techniques of Normalization and Naturalization of Fertility Clinics." In *Reproducing Reproduction: Kinship, Power, and Technological Innovation,* edited by Sarah Franklin and Heléna Ragoné. Philadelphia: University of Pennsylvania Press, 1998.

Dailey, Anne C. "Imagination and Choice." *Law and Social Inquiry* 35, no. 1 (2010): 175–216.

Davis, Boyd H. and Jeutonne P. Brewer. *Electronic Discourse: Linguistic Individuals in Virtual Space.* New York: State University of New York Press, 1997.

Dillman, Ilham. *Love and Human Separateness.* Oxford: Blackwell, 1987.

Dworkin, Andrea. *Right-Wing Women.* London: Women's Press, 1987.

Eisenberg, Melvin Aron. "The Limits of Cognition and the Limits of Contract." *Stanford Law Review* 47, no. 2 (1995): 211–59.

Eliasoph, Nina and Paul Lichterman. "Culture in Interaction." *American Journal of Sociology* 108, no. 4 (2003): 735–94.

Emerson, Robert M. "Ethnography, Interaction, and Ordinary Trouble." *Ethnography* 10, no. 4 (2009): 535–48.

Emerson, Robert M., Rachel I. Fretz, and Linda L. Shaw. *Writing Ethnographic Fieldnotes.* Chicago: University of Chicago Press, 1995.

Epstein, Richard. "Surrogacy: The Case for Full Contractual Enforcement." *Virginia Law Review* 81, no. 8 (1995): 2305–41.

Espeland, Wendy Nelson and Mitchell L. Stevens. "Commensuration as a Social Process." *Annual Review of Sociology* 24 (1998): 313–43.

Ewick, Patricia and Susan S. Silbey. "Conformity, Contestation, and Resistance: An Account of Legal Consciousness." *New England Law Review* 26 (1992): 731–49.

Fernback, Jan. "There Is a There There: Notes toward a Definition of Cybercommunity." In *Doing Internet Research: Critical Issues and Methods for Examining the Net,* edited by Steve Jones, 203–220. Thousand Oaks, CA: Sage, 1999.

Field, Martha A. *Surrogate Motherhood.* Cambridge, MA: Harvard University Press, 1988.

Fine, Gary A. "The Sociology of the Local: Action and Its Publics." *Sociological Theory* 28, no. 4 (2010): 355–76.

Fourcade, Marion. "Theories of Markets and Theories of Society." *American Behavioral Scientist* 50, no. 8 (2007): 1015–34.

Fourcade, Marion and Kieran Healy. "Moral Views of Market Society." *Annual Review of Sociology* 33 (2007): 285–311.

Fox, Renée C. and Judith P. Swazey. *The Courage to Fail. A Social View of Organ Transplants and Dialysis.* Chicago: University of Chicago Press, 1974.

Frank, Arthur W. *Letting Stories Breathe: A Socio-Narratology.* Chicago: University of Chicago Press, 2010.

———. *The Wounded Storyteller: Body, Illness, and Ethics.* Chicago: University of Chicago Press, 1995.

Franklin, Sarah. "Deconstructing 'Desperateness': The Social Construction of Infertility in Popular Representations of New Reproductive Technologies." In *The New Reproductive Technologies,* edited by Maureen McNeil, Ian Varcoe, and Steven Yearley. New York: St. Martin's Press, 1990.

———. "Making Miracles: Scientific Progress and the Facts of Life." In *Reproducing Reproduction: Kinship, Power, and Technological Innovation,* edited by Sarah Franklin and Heléna Ragoné. Philadelphia: University of Pennsylvania Press, 1998.

———. "Making Representations: The Parliamentary Debate on the Human Fertilisation and Embryology Act." In *Technologies of Procreation: Kinship in the Age of Assisted Conception.* 2nd ed. Edited by Jeanette Edwards, Sarah Franklin, Eric Hirsch, Frances Price, and Marilyn Strathern. New York: Routledge, 1999.

Franklin, Sarah and Heléna Ragoné, eds. *Reproducing Reproduction: Kinship, Power, and Technological Innovation.* Philadelphia: University of Pennsylvania Press, 1998.

Franklin, Sarah and Cecil Roberts. *Born and Made: An Ethnography of Preimplantation Genetic Diagnosis.* Princeton, NJ: Princeton University Press, 2006.

Geertz, Clifford. *Interpretation of Cultures.* New York: Basic Books, 1973.

Gilfoyle, Timothy J. "Prostitutes in History: From Parables of Pornography to Metaphors of Modernity." *American Historical Review* 104, no. 1 (1999): 117–41.

Ginsburg, Faye D. and Rayna Rapp, *Conceiving the New World Order: The Global Politics of Reproduction.* Berkeley: University of California, 1995.

Goffman, Erving. *Interaction Ritual: Essays on Face-to-Face Behavior.* New York: Pantheon Books, 1967.

———. "The Moral Career of the Mental Patient." *Psychiatry: Journal for the Study of Interpersonal Processes* 22, no. 2 (1959): 123–42.

———. "The Nature of Deference and Demeanor." *American Anthropologist* 58, no. 3 (1956): 473–502.

———. *The Presentation of Self in Everyday Life.* New York: Doubleday, 1959.

———. *Relations in Public: Microstudies of the Public Order.* New York: Basic Books, 1971.

———. *Stigma: Notes on the Management of Spoiled Identity.* New York: Simon and Schuster, 1963.

Hadfield, Gillian. "An Expressive Theory of Contract: From Feminist Dilemmas to a Reconceptualization of Rational Choice in Contract Law." *University of Pennsylvania Law Review* 146, no. 5 (1998): 1235–85.

Hardey, Michael. "Doctor in the House: The Internet as a Source of Lay Health Knowledge and the Challenge to Expertise." *Sociology of Health and Illness* 21 (1999): 820–35.

Hartocollis, Anemona. "And Baby Makes 3: In New York, a Push for Compensated Surrogacy." *The New York Times,* 19 February 2014.

Hartouni, Valerie. "Reflections on Abortion Politics and the Practices Called 'Person.'" In *Fetal Subjects, Feminist Positions,* edited by Lynn M. Morgan and Meredith W. Michaels. Philadelphia: University of Pennsylvania Press, 1999.

Haylett, Jennifer. "One Woman Helping Another: Egg Donation as a Case of Relational Work." *Politics and Society* 40, no. 2 (2012): 223–47.

Healy, Kieran. *Last Best Gifts: Altruism and the Market for Human Blood and Organs.* Chicago: University of Chicago Press, 2006.

Hine, Christine. *Virtual Ethnography.* Thousand Oaks, CA: Sage, 2000.

Hinson, Diane and Maureen McBrian. "Surrogacy across America." Accessed 15 September 2013. http://claradoc.gpa.free.fr/doc/431.pdf.

Hooley, Tristram, Jane Wellens, and John Marriott. *What Is Online Research? Using the Internet for Social Science Research.* London: Bloomsbury Academic, 2012.

Hughes, Everett C. *On Work, Race, and the Sociological Imagination.* Chicago: University of Chicago Press, 1994.

Illouz, Eva. *Consuming the Romantic Utopia: Love and the Cultural Contradictions of Capitalism.* Berkeley: University of California Press, 1997.

Inhorn, Marcia C. *Local Babies, Global Science: Gender, Religion, and in Vitro Fertilization in Egypt.* New York: Routledge, 2003.

Inhorn, Marcia C. and Daphna Birenbaum-Carmeli. "Assisted Reproductive Technologies and Cultural Change." *Annual Review of Anthropology* 37 (2008): 177–96.

Inhorn, Marcia and Frank van Balen, eds. *Infertility around the Globe. New Thinking on Childlessness, Gender, and Reproductive Technologies.* Berkeley: University of California Press, 2002.

Isaacson, Nicole F. "The 'Fetus-Infant': Changing Classifications of in Utero Development in Medical Texts." *Sociological Forum* 11, no. 3 (1996): 457–80.

Jenkins, Richard. *Social Identity.* New York: Routledge, 1996.

Jones, Steve. "Studying the Net: Intricacies and Issues." In *Doing Internet Research: Critical Issues and Methods for Examining the Net.* Thousand Oaks, CA: Sage, 1999.

Jones, Steven G. "Information, Internet, and Community: Notes toward an Understanding of Community in the Information Age." In *Cybersociety 2.0: Revisiting Computer-Mediated Communication and Community.* Thousand Oaks, CA: Sage, 1998.

Kapferer, Bruce. "Emotion and Feeling in Singhalese Healing Rites." *Social Analysis* 1 (1979): 153–73.

Katz, Jack. "Ethnography's Warrants." *Sociological Methods and Research* 25, no. 4 (1997): 391–423.

———. "From How to Why: On Luminous Description and Causal Inference in Ethnography (Part I)." *Ethnography* 2, no. 4 (2001): 443–73.

Kendall, Lori. "Recontextualizing Cyberspace: Methodological Consider-ations for On-line Research." In *Doing Internet Research: Critical Issues and Methods for Examining the Net,* edited by Steve Jones. Thousand Oaks, CA: Sage, 1999.

Kerian, Christine. "Surrogacy: A Last Resort Alternative for Infertile Women or a Commodification of Women's Bodies and Children?" *Wisconsin Women's Law Journal* 12, no. 1 (1997): 113–66.

Ketchum, Sara A. "Selling Babies and Selling Bodies." In *Feminist Perspectives in Medical Ethics,* edited by H. Bequaert Holmes and L.M. Purdy, 264–94. Bloomington: Indiana University Press, 1992.

Klaus, Marshall H. and John H. Kennell. *Maternal-Infant Bonding: The Impact of Early Separation or Loss on Family Development.* St-Louis: Mosby, 1976.

Konrad, Monica. *Nameless Relations: Anonymity, Melanesia, and Reproductive Gift Exchange between British Ova Donors and Recipients.* New York: Berghahn, 2005.

Kopytoff, Igor. "The Cultural Biography of Things: Commoditization as Process." In *The Social Life of Things: Commodities in Cultural Perspective,* edited by A. Appadurai. Cambridge: Cambridge University Press, 1986.

Krawiec, Kimberly D. "Altruism and Intermediation in the Market for Babies." *Washington and Lee Law Review* 66 (2009): 1–55.

Lakoff, George and Mark Johnson. *Metaphors We Live By.* Chicago: University of Chicago Press, 2008.

Lareau, Annette. *Unequal Childhoods: Class, Race, and Family Life.* Berkeley: University of California Press, 2003.

Lauritzen, Paul. *Pursuing Parenthood: Ethical Issues in Assisted Reproduction.* Bloomington: Indiana University Press, 1993.

Layne, Linda L. *Motherhood Lost. A Feminist Account of Pregnancy Loss in America.* New York: Routledge, 2003.

———. "'He was a Real Baby with Baby Things' A Material Culture Analysis of Personhood, Parenthood and Pregnancy Loss." *Journal of Material Culture* 5, no. 3 (2000): 321-345.

Levine, Hal B. "Gestational Surrogacy: Nature and Culture in Kinship." *Ethnology* 42 (2003): 173–85.

Linde, Charlotte. "Explanatory Systems in Oral Life Stories." In *Cultural Models in Language and Thought,* edited by Dorothy Holland and Naomi Quinn, 343–66. Cambridge: University of Cambridge Press, 1987.

Luker, Kristin. *Dubious Conceptions: The Politics of Teenage Pregnancy.* Cambridge, MA: Harvard University Press, 1996.

Lystra, Karen. *Searching the Heart: Women, Men, and Romantic Love in Nineteenth-Century America.* New York: Oxford University Press, 1989.

MacDonald, Kerri. "Letting Go of a Baby, but Not the Emotions." *New York Times,* 10 May 2013.

Madge, Clare and Henrietta O'Connor. "Parenting Gone Wired: Empowerment of New Mothers on the Internet?" *Social & Cultural Geography* 7, no. 2 (2006): 199–220.

Mamo, Laura. *Queering Reproduction: Achieving Pregnancy in the Age of Tech-noscience*. Durham: Duke University Press, 2007.

Mann, Chris and Fiona Stewart. *Internet Communication and Qualitative Research: A Handbook for Researching Online*. Thousand Oaks, CA: Sage, 2000.

Markens, Susan. "The Global Reproductive Health Market: U.S. Media Framings and Public Discourses about Transnational Surrogacy." *Social Science & Medicine* 74, no. 11 (2012): 1745–53.

———. "Interrogating Narratives about the Global Surrogacy Market." *The Scholar and Feminist Online* 9, nos. 1–2 (2011). http://sfonline.barnard.edu/reprotech/markens_01.htm.

———. *Surrogate Motherhood and the Politics of Reproduction*. Berkeley: University of California Press, 2007.

Markens, Susan, Carole H. Browner, and H. Mabel Preloran. "Interrogating the Dynamics between Power, Knowledge and Pregnant Bodies in Amniocentesis Decision Making." *Sociology of Health & Illness* 32, no. 1 (2010): 37–56.

Mattingly, Charyl. *Healing Dramas and Clinical Plots: The Narrative Structure of Experience*. Cambridge: Cambridge University Press, 1998.

Mauss, Marcel. *The Gift: The Form and Reason for Exchange in Archaic Societies*. New York: W.W. Norton, 1990.

McLachlan, Hugh V. and Kim Swales. "Commercial Surrogate Motherhood and the Alleged Commodification of Children: A Defense of Legally Enforceable Contracts." *Law and Contemporary Problems* 72 (2009): 91–107.

Mills, C. Wright. "Situated Actions and Vocabularies of Motive." *American Sociological Review* 5 (1940): 904–13.

Mitchell, Lisa Meryn. *Baby's First Picture: Ultrasound and the Politics of Fetal Subjects*. Toronto: University of Toronto Press, 2001.

Ortner, Sherry B. "Introduction." *Representations* 59 (1997): 1–13.

Overall, Christine. *Ethics and Human Reproduction: A Feminist Analysis*. Boston: Allen and Unwin, 1987.

Pande, Amrita. "'It May Be Her Eggs but It's My Blood': Surrogates and Everyday Forms of Kinship in India." *Qualitative Sociology* 32, no. 4 (2009): 379–97.

———. "Not an 'Angel', not a 'Whore': Surrogates as 'Dirty' Workers in India." *Indian Journal of Gender Studies* 16, no. 2 (2009): 141–73.

———. *Wombs in Labor: Transnational Commercial Surrogacy in India*. New York: Columbia University Press, 2014.

Park, Robert E. *Race and Culture*. Glencoe, IL: Free Press, 1950.

Parry, Jonathan. "The Gift, the Indian Gift, and the 'Indian Gift.'" *Man* 21, no. 3 (1986): 453–73.

Parry, Jonathan and Maurice Bloch, eds. *Money and the Morality of Exchange*. New York: Cambridge University Press, 1989.

Peletz, Michael G. "Kinship Studies in Late Twentieth-Century Anthropology." *Annual Review of Anthropology* 24 (1995): 343–72.

Pitts, Victoria. "Illness and Internet Empowerment: Writing and Reading Breast Cancer in Cyberspace." *Health* 8, no. 1 (2004): 33–59.

Pollner, Melvin. "Mundane Reasoning." *Philosophy of the Social Sciences* 4, no. 1 (1974): 35–54.

Pollner, Melvin and Jill Stein. "Narrative Mapping of Social Worlds: The Voice of Experience in Alcoholics Anonymous." *Symbolic Interaction* 19, no. 3 (1996): 203–23.

Posner, Richard A. "The Ethics and Economics of Enforcing Contracts of Surrogate Motherhood." *Journal of Contemporary Health Law and Policy* 5 (1989): 21.

Prasad, Monica. "The Morality of Market Exchange: Love, Money, and Contractual Justice." *Sociological Perspectives* 42 (1999): 181–213.

Purdy, Laura M. *Reproducing Persons: Issues in Feminist Bioethics.* Ithaca, NY: Cornell University Press, 1996.

Radin, Margaret Jane. *Contested Commodities: The Trouble with Trade in Sex, Children, Body Parts, and Other Things.* Cambridge, MA: Harvard University Press, 1996.

———. "Market-Inalienability," *Harvard Law Review* 100, no. 8 (1987): 1849–937.

———. "What, If Anything, Is Wrong with Baby Selling?" *Pacific Law Review* 26, no. 2 (1995): 135–45.

Radin, Patricia. "'To Me, It's My Life': Medical Communication, Trust, and Activism in Cyberspace." *Social Science & Medicine* 62, no. 3 (2006): 591–601.

Ragoné, Heléna. "The Gift of Life." In *Transformative Motherhood: On Giving and Getting in a Consumer Culture,* edited by Linda L. Layne. New York: New York University Press, 1999.

———. "Incontestable Motivations." In *Reproducing Reproduction: Kinship, Power, and Technological Innovation,* edited by S. Franklin and H. Ragoné. Philadelphia: University of Pennsylvania Press, 1998.

———. *Surrogate Motherhood: Conceptions in the Heart.* Boulder, CO: Westview, 1994.

Rapp, Rayna. *Testing Women, Testing the Fetus. The Social Impact of Amniocentesis in America.* New York: Routledge, 1999.

Reading, A.E. and J.F. Kerin. "Psychological Aspects of Providing Infertility Services." *Journal of Reproductive Medicine* 34 (1989): 861–71.

Reddy, William M. *The Navigation of Feeling. A Framework for the History of Emotions.* Cambridge: Cambridge University Press, 2001.

Rheingold, Howard. *The Virtual Community: Homesteading on the Electronic Frontier.* Cambridge, MA: MIT Press, 2000.

Roberts, Elizabeth F.S. "Examining Surrogacy Discourses between Feminine Power and Exploitation." In *Small Wars: The Cultural Politics of Childhood,* edited by N. Scheper-Hughes and C. Sargent, 93–110. Berkeley: University of California Press, 1998.

———. *God's Laboratory. Assisted Reproduction in the Andes.* Berkeley: University of California Press, 2012.

———. "'Native' Narratives of Connectedness: Surrogate Motherhood and Technology." In *Cyborg Babies: From Techno-Sex to Techno-Tots,* edited by R. Davis-Floyd and J. Dumit. New York: Routledge, 1998.

Roberts, Melinda A. "Good Intentions and a Great Divide: Having Babies by Intending Them." *Law and Philosophy* 12, no. 3 (1993): 287–317.

Robertson, John. *Children of Choice: Freedom and the New Reproductive Technologies.* Princeton, NJ: Princeton University Press, 1994.

Robinson, Laura and Jeremy Schulz. "New Avenues for Sociological Inquiry: Evolving Forms of Ethnographic Practice." *Sociology* 43, no. 4 (2009): 685–98.

Rose, Nikolas and Carlos Novas. "Biological Citizenship." http://thesp.leeds. ac.uk/files/2014/04/RoseandNovasBiologicalCitizenship2002.pdf.

Rothman, Barbara Katz. "Comment on Harrison: The Commodification of Motherhood." *Gender and Society* 1, no. 3 (1987): 312–16.

———. *Recreating Motherhood.* New York: W.W. Norton, 1989.

———. "Reproductive Technology and the Commodification of Life." In *Embryos, Ethics, and Women's Rights,* edited by E.H. Baruch, A.F. D'Adamo, Jr., and J. Seager. New York: Haworth Press, 1988.

———. "Women as Fathers: Motherhood and Child Care under a Modified Patriarchy." *Gender & Society* 3, no. 1 (1989): 89–104.

Rudrappa, Sharmila. "India's Reproductive Assembly Line." *Contexts* 11, no. 2 (2012): 22–27.

Sandel, Michael J. "What Money Can't Buy: The Moral Limits of the Market." The Tanner Lecture on Human Values. 2000. Accessed August 12, 2005. http://74.125.155.132/scholar?q=cache:R723YTlN-lYJ:scholar. google.com/+sandel+michael+2000&hl=en&as_sdt=2000.

Sandelowski, Margarete. *With Child in Mind: Studies of the Personal Encounter with Infertility.* Philadelphia: University of Pennsylvania Press, 1993.

Saul, Stephanie. "Building a Baby, with Few Ground Rules." *The New York Times,* December 12, 2009.

Sawicki, Jana. *Disciplining Foucault: Feminism, Power, and the Body.* New York: Routledge, 1991.

Scheper-Hughes, Nancy. *Death without Weeping: The Violence of Everyday Life in Brazil.* Berkeley: University of California Press, 1993.

Schmidtz, David. "Reasons for Altruism." *Social Philosophy and Policy* 10, no. 1 (1993): 52–68.

Schneider, David M. *American Kinship: A Cultural Account.* Englewood Cliffs, NJ: Prentice-Hall, 1968.

Schneider, David M. and Raymond T. Smith. *Class Differences in American Kinship.* Ann Arbor: University of Michigan Press, 1978.

Schuck, Peter. "Some Reflections on the Baby M Case." *Georgetown Law Journal* 76, no. 5 (1987): 1793–810.

Schwartz, Loretta L. "Surrogacy Arrangements in the USA: What Relationships Do They Spawn?" In *Surrogate Motherhood: International Perspectives,* edited by Rachel Cook, Shelley Day Sclater, and Felicity Kaganas. Oxford: Hart, 2003.

Scott, Elizabeth S. "Surrogacy and the Politics of Commodification." *Law and Contemporary Problems* 72 (2009): 109–46.

Seale, Clive. "Gender Accommodation in Online Cancer Support Groups." *Health* 10, no. 3 (2006): 345–60.

Sewell, William H., Jr. 1999. "The Concept(s) of Culture." In *Beyond the Cultural Turn: New Directions in the Study of Society and Culture,* edited by V.E. Bonnell and L. Hunt. Berkeley: University of California Press, 1999.

Shalev, Carmel. *Birth Power: A Case for Surrogacy.* New Haven, CT: Yale University Press, 1989.

Shanley, Mary L. *Making Babies, Making Families.* Boston: Beacon, 2001.

———. "'Surrogate Mothering' and Women's Freedom: A Critique of Contracts for Human Reproduction." *Signs* 18, no. 3 (1993): 618–39.

Sharf, Barbara F. "Communicating Breast Cancer On-line: Support and Empowerment on the Internet." *Women and Health* 26, no. 1 (1997): 65–84.

Sharp, Lesley A. "Organ Transplantation as a Transformative Experience: Anthropological Insights into the Restructuring of the Self." *Medical Anthropology Quarterly* 9, no. 3 (1995): 357–89.

Simmel, Georg. "Faithfulness and Gratitude." In *The Sociology of Georg Simmel,* edited by K.H. Wolff, 379–95. New York: Free Press, 1950.

———. *The Philosophy of Money.* Translated by Tom Bottomore and David Frisby. London: Routledge and Kegan Paul, 1978.

Solomon, Robert. *About Love: Reinventing Romance for Our Times.* New York: Simon and Schuster, 1988.

Stack, Carol B. *All Our Kin: Strategies for Survival in a Black Community.* New York: Basic Books, 1975.

Strasser, Mark. "Tradition Surrogacy Contracts, Partial Enforcement, and the Challenge for Family Law." *Journal of Health Care Law & Policy,* 18 (2015): 85-113.

Strathern, Marilyn. "Partners and Consumers: Making Relations Visible." In *The Logic of the Gift: Toward an Ethic of Generosity,* edited by Alan D. Schrift, 292–311. New York: Routledge, 1997.

———. *Reproducing the Future: Essays on Anthropology, Kinship, and the New Reproductive Technologies.* New York: Routledge, 1992.

Taft, Lee. "Apology Subverted: The Commodification of Apology." *Yale Law Journal* 109, no. 5 (2000): 1135–60.

Tavory, Iddo and Stefan Timmermans. "Two Cases of Ethnography: Grounded Theory and the Extended Case Method." *Ethnography* 10, no. 3 (2009): 243–63.

Taylor, Janelle S. *The Public Life of the Fetal Sonogram: Technology, Consumption, and the Politics of Reproduction.* New Brunswick, NJ: Rutgers University Press, 2008.

Teman, Elly. *Birthing a Mother: The Surrogate Body and the Pregnant Self.* Berkeley: University of California Press, 2010.

———. "'Knowing' the Surrogate Body in Israel." In *Surrogate Motherhood: International Perspectives,* edited by Rachel Cook, Shelley Day Sclater, and Felicity Kaganas. Oxford: Hart, 2003.

Teman, Elly. "The Social Construction of Surrogacy Research: An Anthropological Critique of the Psychosocial Scholarship on Surrogate Motherhood." *Social Science and Medicine* 67 (2008): 104–12.

Thompson, Charis. *Making Parents. The Ontological Choreography of Reproductive Technologies.* Cambridge, MA: MIT Press, 2005.

Tilly, Charles. *Why? What Happens When People Give Reasons . . . and Why.* Princeton, NJ: Princeton University Press, 2006.

Turkle, Sherry. "Cyberspace and Identity." *Contemporary Sociology* 28, no. 6 (1999): 643–48.

Twine, France Winddance. *Outsourcing the Womb: Race, Class and Gestational Surrogacy in a Global Market.* New York: Routledge, 2015.

Virnoche, Mary and Gary Marx. "'Only Connect'—E.M. Forster in an Age of Electronic Communication: Computer-Mediated Association and Community Networks." *Sociological Inquiry* 67 (1997): 85–100.

Vora, Kalindi. "Potential, Risk, and Return in Transnational Indian Gestational Surrogacy." *Current Anthropology* 54, no. S7 (2013): S97–S106.

Williams, Raymond. *Keywords: A Vocabulary of Culture and Society.* New York: Oxford University Press, 1985.

Wittel, Andreas. "Ethnography on the Move: From Field to Net to Internet." *Forum: Qualitative Social Research* 1, no. 1 (2000). http://www.qualitative-research.net/index.php/fqs/article/view/1131/2517.

Wuthnow, Robert. *Meaning and Moral Order.* Berkeley: University of California Press, 1987.

Yngvesson, Barbara. "Placing the 'Gift Child' in Transnational Adoption." *Law and Society Review* 36 (2002): 227–56.

Zelizer, Viviana A. "How I Became a Relational Economic Sociologist and What Does That Mean?" *Politics & Society* 40, no. 2 (2012): 145–74.

———. "Human Values and the Market: The Case of Life Insurance and Death in 19th-Century America." *American Journal of Sociology* 84, no. 3 (1978): 591–610.

———. "Love's Hikers Don't Walk Alone." *Newsletter of the Sociology of Culture* 18 (2004): 3–4.

———. "Monetization and Social Life." *Etnofoor* 13, no. 2 (2000): 5–15.

———. "Payments and Social Ties." *Sociological Forum* 11 (1996): 481–95.

———. *Pricing the Priceless Child: The Changing Social Value of Children.* Princeton, NJ: Princeton University Press, 1985.

———. *The Purchase of Intimacy.* Princeton, NJ: Princeton University Press, 2005.

———. *The Social Meaning of Money.* New York: Basic Books, 1994.

Index

Fertility, Reproduction and Sexuality

GENERAL EDITORS:

Soraya Tremayne, Founding Director, Fertility and Reproduction Studies Group, and Research Associate, Institute of Social and Cultural Anthropology, University of Oxford.

Marcia C. Inhorn, William K. Lanman, Jr. Professor of Anthropology and International Affairs, Yale University.

Philip Kreager, Director, Fertility and Reproduction Studies Group, and Research Associate, Institute of Social and Cultural Anthropology and Institute of Human Sciences, University of Oxford.